Fast Facts

Asthma

Third edition

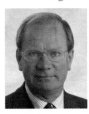

Stephen T Holgate MD DSc FRCP FMedSci
MRC Clinical Professor of Immunopharmacology
School of Medicine
Southampton General Hospital
Southampton, UK

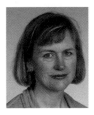

Jo Douglass MB BS MD FRACP
Head, Allergy, Asthma and Clinical
Immunology Service
Alfred Hospital and Monash University
Melbourne, Victoria, Australia

Declaration of Independence
This book is as balanced and as practical as we can make it.
Ideas for improvement are always welcome: feedback@fastfacts.com

Fast Facts: Asthma
First published 1999
Second edition 2006; reprinted 2007
Third edition January 2010

Text © 2010 Stephen T Holgate, Jo Douglass
© 2010 in this edition Health Press Limited
Health Press Limited, Elizabeth House, Queen Street, Abingdon,
Oxford OX14 3LN, UK
Tel: +44 (0)1235 523233
Fax: +44 (0)1235 523238

Book orders can be placed by telephone or via the website.
For regional distributors or to order via the website, please go to: www.fastfacts.com
For telephone orders, please call 01752 202301 (UK), +44 1752 202301 (Europe),
1 800 247 6553 (USA, toll free), +1 419 281 1802 (Americas) or
+61 (0)2 9698 7755 (Asia–Pacific).

Fast Facts is a trademark of Health Press Limited.

A CIP record for this title is available from the British Library.

ISBN 978-1-905832-66-8

Holgate ST (Stephen)
Fast Facts: Asthma/
Stephen T Holgate, Jo Douglass

Medical illustrations by Dee McLean and Jane Fallows,
London, UK.
Typesetting and page layout by Zed, Oxford, UK.
Printed by Latimer Trend & Company, Plymouth, UK.

Text printed on biodegradable and recyclable paper
manufactured using elemental chlorine free (ECF) wood
pulp from well-managed forests.

FSC

Mixed Sources
Product group from well-managed
forests and other controlled sources

Cert no. SGS-COC-005493
www.fsc.org
© 1996 Forest Stewardship Council

Glossary

AMP: adenosine 5'-monophosphate

ASA: acetylsalicylic acid (aspirin)

Atopy: a condition characterized by excessive production of immunoglobulin (Ig)E in response to allergens

Basophil: a type of white blood cell, distinguishable on staining

B lymphocyte: a type of white blood cell that produces antibodies

COPD: chronic obstructive pulmonary disease

CysLTs: cysteinyl leukotrienes, a powerful class of bronchoconstricting mediators

Cytokine: a peptide secreted by cells involved in inflammation and the immune response; cytokines can control the activity and growth of the cell that secreted them, or nearby cells

Daily variability: variability in daily peak expiratory flow (PEF), calculated as a percentage of the mean daily PEF value

DPI: dry-powder inhaler

Eosinophil: a type of white blood cell involved in allergic responses, distinguishable on staining

FEV$_1$: forced expiratory volume in 1 second, a measure of lung function

FVC: forced vital capacity, a measure of lung function

GINA: Global Initiative for Asthma, an international scientific initiative created to provide and encourage the use of scientific reports on asthma and asthma research

IFNγ: interferon-γ, a cytokine that has the capacity to inhibit the development of the allergic pathways, under normal conditions

IgE: immunoglobulin class E, a class of antibody secreted by B lymphocytes on exposure to allergen; binding of IgE to certain cells involved in the immune response results in the release of inflammatory mediators

IL: interleukin, a cytokine that controls a specific aspect of hemopoiesis or the immune response

LABA: long-acting β$_2$-agonist

Leukocyte: white blood cell

Mast cell: a large cell containing chemical mediators that are released in inflammatory and allergic responses

MDI: metered-dose inhaler

NSAID: non-steroidal anti-inflammatory drug

PaCO$_2$: partial pressure of carbon dioxide in arterial blood

PaO$_2$: partial pressure of oxygen in arterial blood

PEF: peak expiratory flow, a measure of lung function

pMDI: pressurized metered-dose inhaler

SABA: short-acting β$_2$-agonist

SpO$_2$: oxygen saturation measured by pulse oximeter

T lymphocyte: a type of white blood cell that is mainly responsible for cell-mediated immunity

Th lymphocyte: T helper lymphocyte; a type of T lymphocyte that is activated on exposure to allergen and releases cytokines

Trigger: a stimulus that increases asthma symptoms and/or airflow limitation

Introduction

Asthma remains a major cause of morbidity and mortality throughout the world. This involves not only the burden of disease to individuals through loss of life and hospital admissions, but also in lost productivity as asthma remains a leading cause of absences from work and school. Whilst asthma mortality in developed nations appears to be stable or declining, international studies still report a very high burden of illness in those with asthma despite the availability of very effective asthma treatments.

It has long been recognized that asthma is a disorder of widespread airway obstruction, reversible either spontaneously or with treatment. It is also clear that underlying airway inflammation is a predominant cause of airway dysfunction in asthma, leading to increased responsiveness to a variety of stimuli. Recent research has identified some of the fundamental immunologic and cellular differences of the asthmatic airway, leading to greater understanding of the chronic inflammation associated with accelerated loss of lung function, which is characteristic of asthma.

Asthma most commonly begins in early childhood, but may occur in any age group and persist through life. Recent large epidemiological studies have identified several groups of very young children who wheeze, not all of whom will have asthma. However, once asthma is established, its severity, like all chronic inflammatory diseases, may vary from mild and intermittent to severe and persistent. Thus, its impact on the quality of life of an individual can vary greatly. However, if asthma is correctly diagnosed and properly treated, most patients can lead a normal life, although many will need to take medications regularly.

Because of the chronic nature of asthma, its underlying airway abnormalities and the burden of disease, national and international guidelines for asthma management have been developed that focus on:
- accurate asthma diagnosis
- objective assessment of airway inflammation and its severity
- prevention of asthma with drug treatment
- patient education

- management strategies
- monitoring.

This fully updated third edition of *Fast Facts: Asthma* draws its treatment recommendations from the Global Initiative for Asthma (GINA) guidelines, produced by the World Health Organization and the US National Heart Lung and Blood Institute and based on best available evidence. Key to these guidelines is the prescription of asthma treatments, which is determined by the level of asthma symptoms requiring control. In this book we have attempted to distill the essential features of the latest GINA treatment guidelines into a palatable and easily accessible form without losing information.

By the time guidelines for any disease are written and published they are, almost by definition, out of date on account of the continued research into the disease and its management. Asthma is no exception. It is our intention that this book provides the basis for good asthma management. However, guidelines are guidelines, and should not be taken as rules. The individual patient must be assessed in his or her own right, with individual circumstances taken into account. The principles raised in this book should nevertheless provide a framework to improve the lives of the many patients with this disease.

Asthma is a chronic inflammatory condition of the airways. It is characterized by recurrent episodes of airflow limitation which, depending on the severity of the attack, produce symptoms such as breathlessness, wheezing, chest tightness and cough. Acute exacerbations can be rapid or gradual in onset, and may be severe and potentially life-threatening.

Autopsy studies of patients who have died from asthma show hyperinflated lungs, with both large and small airways blocked by plugs containing a mixture of mucus, serum proteins, inflammatory cells and cell debris. Microscopic examination reveals extensive inflammatory infiltration of the airways (Figure 1.1), with edema due to vasodilatation

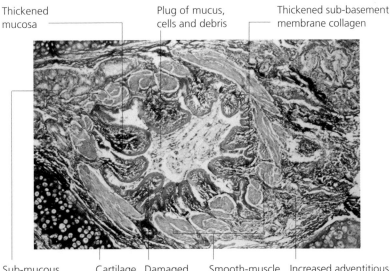

Figure 1.1 Pathological features associated with death from asthma. Airways are blocked by plugs of mucus and inflammatory exudate. There is also vasodilatation and edema, vascular remodeling, smooth muscle hypertrophy and thickening of the basement membrane.

and blood vessel engorgement, and epithelial disruption. Biopsy studies have shown increased numbers of leukocytes, particularly eosinophils, mast cells and T lymphocytes, in the airways, and increases in the markers of lymphocyte activation. Structural changes resulting from chronic inflammation include bronchial smooth muscle hypertrophy and hyperplasia, new vessel formation, interstitial collagen deposition resulting in basement membrane thickening, and airway wall remodeling.

Disease mechanisms

In many cases, asthma is an allergic disorder mediated in part by immunoglobulin (Ig)E-dependent mechanisms. Exposure to allergen results in allergen uptake and its presentation by dendritic cells to T helper (Th) lymphocytes (Figure 1.2).

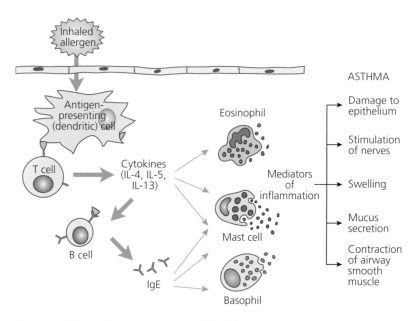

Figure 1.2 Role of immunoglobulin E (IgE) in airway inflammation and asthma symptoms. Exposure to allergen leads to activation of T lymphocytes, cytokine expression (interleukins [ILs]) and release of IgE from B lymphocytes. IgE binds to cells involved in inflammation, which then release inflammatory mediators.

Th lymphocytes are categorized according to the dominant pattern of cytokines secreted. Those secreting interleukin (IL)-4, IL-5 and IL-13 are Th2, and stimulate the production of IgE from B lymphocytes. Conversely, Th1 lymphocytes produce interferon-γ (IFNγ), which facilitates the secretion of IgG by B lymphocytes. T lymphocytes in asthmatic epithelium predominantly release a Th2 pattern of cytokines, indicating the cardinal importance of Th2 lymphocytes in driving the eosinophilic inflammation that is characteristic of asthma.

The IgE produced by the stimulated B lymphocytes binds to mast cells and, possibly, other cells involved in inflammation (e.g. eosinophils), leading to the release of inflammatory mediators. Further exposure to antigens can also provoke T-cell activation, cytokine and chemokine release, and production of inflammatory mediators by IgE-independent mechanisms.

Chronic inflammation is responsible for the two principal manifestations of disordered lung function in asthma: bronchial hyperresponsiveness and acute limitation of airflow (Table 1.1). Patients with asthma show an enhanced bronchoconstrictive response to a variety of stimuli such as histamine and methacholine (which act directly on airway smooth muscle), and exercise, adenosine 5'-monophosphate (AMP) and cold or dry air (which act indirectly), causing airway narrowing secondary to the release of inflammatory mediators.

TABLE 1.1

Manifestations of disordered lung function in asthma

- Airway hyperresponsiveness
- Airflow limitation
  - acute bronchoconstriction
  - swelling of the airway wall
  - chronic mucus plug formation
  - airway wall remodeling
- Stimulation of neurons
  - cough
  - chest tightness

Airway diameter becomes more variable, as reflected by variation in measures of lung function such as peak expiratory flow (PEF; Figure 1.3). Characteristically in asthma, PEF varies by more than 20% between morning and evening measurements.

In asthmatic airways, reductions in airflow can be due to acute bronchoconstriction, swelling of the airway wall, chronic mucous plugging or airway wall remodeling. Acute bronchoconstriction may occur as a result of allergen-induced release of inflammatory mediators

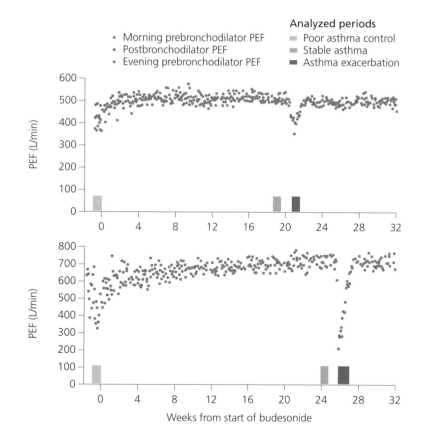

Figure 1.3 Peak expiratory flow (PEF), with and without budesonide treatment, showing within-day and between-day variations and exacerbations for 2 patients. Reproduced from Reddel et al. *Lancet* 1999;353:364–9 with permission from Elsevier.

such as histamine, prostaglandins and leukotrienes. Swelling of the airway wall is caused by edema, with or without bronchoconstriction. Chronic inflammation can also lead to hypersecretion of mucus and exudation, resulting in plugging of the airways and, ultimately, matrix deposition and airway remodeling (see Figure 1.1).

Definition of asthma based on pathophysiology

An operational definition of asthma in which symptoms are related to the underlying pathophysiology (Table 1.2) has important consequences for diagnosis and treatment. Repeating lung function measurements to take account of the marked variation in airflow in asthma is an important element in the diagnosis (see Chapter 3). Similarly, recognition that asthma is a chronic inflammatory disorder has focused attention on the use of corticosteroids in long-term management (see Chapter 4).

While historically asthma has been defined as a disease characterized by the presence of eosinophils in mucosal inflammation, examination of induced sputum cell counts has defined some forms of asthma that appear to be associated with non-eosinophilic inflammation. These types of asthma have been defined as neutrophilic and paucigranulocytic (in which there is a normal cellular profile). In contrast to the apparently corticosteroid-responsive eosinophilic/Th2 cytokine inflammatory

---

TABLE 1.2

An operational definition of asthma based on underlying pathophysiology

- Asthma is a chronic inflammatory disorder of the airways, in which many cells and cellular elements play a role

- The chronic inflammation causes an associated increase in airway hyperresponsiveness that leads to recurrent episodes of wheezing, breathlessness, chest tightness and cough, particularly at night and/or in the early morning

- Episodes of asthma symptoms are usually associated with widespread but variable airflow obstruction that is often reversible, either spontaneously or with treatment

pathways, the non-eosinophilic inflammatory pathways are associated with relative corticosteroid resistance. In individual cases, the definition of the asthmatic inflammatory phenotype is being used to guide therapy, especially for asthma that has proven refractory to usual treatment.

Risk factors for asthma

Asthma is a complex condition, and its causes are not fully understood. Risk factors can be categorized as:

- host factors that predispose an individual to asthma
- causal factors, which are environmental factors that influence susceptibility to the development of asthma in predisposed individuals
- trigger factors, which are environmental factors that precipitate asthma exacerbations and/or cause symptoms to persist.

Examples of these factors are shown in Table 1.3. In any given individual, the development of asthma, and the occurrence of acute exacerbations, will be due to an interaction between numerous predisposing, environmental and occupational factors.

Predisposing factors. The most important factor predisposing to asthma is atopy, which is characterized by excessive IgE production in response to allergens. The prevalence of asthma increases with increasing serum IgE concentration; the majority of asthma patients (other than those who develop the condition late in life) are atopic and, in particular, express IgE directed to inhaled allergens. Atopic diseases such as asthma tend to run in families, with heritability accounting for up to 50% of the clinical expression.

Childhood asthma is more common in boys than in girls until the age of about 10 years, when the difference disappears. Severe persistent asthma in adults is more frequent in women. There is some evidence that these differences are due to differences in allergen sensitivity and airway responsiveness between the sexes, although the differential effects of hormones at puberty may also lead to changes in asthma prevalence.

Genetics. Clearly, genetic influences can modify the risk of an individual developing atopy and asthma. While no single gene has been

TABLE 1.3

Potential risk factors for the development or exacerbation of asthma

Predisposing factors

- Genetic predisposition
- Atopy
- Airway hyperresponsiveness
- Sex
- Race/ethnicity
- Family size

Causal factors

- Indoor allergens (domestic mites, animal allergens, cockroach allergen, fungi)
- Outdoor allergens (pollens, fungi)
- Occupational sensitizers
- Tobacco smoking (passive and active)
- Air pollution (outdoor and indoor)
- Respiratory infections
- Parasitic infections
- Socioeconomic status
- Diet and drugs
- Obesity

Trigger factors

- Allergens
- Pollutants
- Respiratory infections
- Exercise and hyperventilation
- Changes in the weather
- Sulfur dioxide
- Foods, additives, drugs
- Extreme emotional expression
- Tobacco smoking
- Irritants (e.g. household sprays, paint fumes)

identified as being causative for asthma, several genetic loci have been associated with increased asthma risk. It is likely that several of these may work synergistically to cause asthma in individuals exposed to appropriate environmental factors. In particular, variants of the genes *ADAM33*, *PHF11*, *HLA-G*, *NPSR1* (also known as *GPRA* and *GPR154*), *IRAK3* (also known as *IRAK-M*) and *ORMDL3* appear to be associated with an increased risk of asthma.

Hygiene hypothesis. A rise in the worldwide prevalence of asthma and allergic diseases has been documented in the past 2 decades, particularly in nations with a Western lifestyle. This rise has been particularly well described in Eastern European countries where the epidemiological findings of a rise in the prevalence of allergy and asthma have been associated with changes in lifestyle such as newer housing and increasing in-home childcare.

In addition, a lower prevalence of asthma has been observed in children raised in a rural environment, suggesting that factors such as degree of exposure to bacterial lipopolysaccharide or alterations in gastrointestinal flora may be important.

The finding that childhood infections such as tuberculosis and hepatitis may be protective for allergy and asthma suggested the 'hygiene hypothesis'. This attributes the rising prevalence of asthma and allergic diseases to a failure of early immune maturation caused by the relative protection from bacterial exposure in the first few years of life that a Western lifestyle offers. Lack of bacterial stimulation of the immature immune system is thought to skew the immune system to produce IgE rather than IgG in response to common allergens.

More recently, it has been observed that the prevalence of some other autoimmune diseases, including juvenile diabetes mellitus and Crohn's disease, has also risen. The hygiene hypothesis has therefore been modified to suggest that failure of bacterial immune stimulation early in life leads to altered maturation of immunoregulatory pathways through T suppressor cells. Further understanding of immune maturation is necessary before the networks involved can be fully traced, but the hypothesis has led to the identification of some areas that show promise for the development of preventive asthma interventions.

Dysfunction of the airway epithelium. In addition to immunologic abnormalities leading to asthma, recent findings also point to a fundamental abnormality in asthmatic airway epithelium as a major factor in generating chronic airway inflammation. Dysfunction of the airway epithelial tight junctions leads to greater permeability of the airway surfaces to inhaled particles, enabling these particles to penetrate the epithelial barrier and to elicit inflammatory responses by contact with inflammatory cells and subepithelial neural pathways.

In addition, the asthmatic epithelium responds to oxidant stress and pathogenic stimulation differently from the non-asthmatic epithelium, producing interferons that lead to increased susceptibility to airway viral infections. These properties, unique to asthmatic epithelium, predispose the asthmatic airway to a more chronic and persistent inflammatory response than would occur in the normal airway.

Causal factors. The relevance of different causes of asthma depends on individual exposure and when it occurs. In early childhood, inhaled allergens and infection appear to be important causal factors for asthma. In adults, cigarette smoking and exposure to occupational allergens are more likely to be important causal factors.

Inhaled allergens. Common indoor sources of inhaled allergens include domestic mites, cats, dogs and fungi. Outdoor pollens from grasses, trees and wind-pollinated weeds are also common inhaled allergens. Allergen exposure leads to the activation of specific T lymphocytes and the production of specific IgE by B lymphocytes, which sensitizes the individual to subsequent exposure. There is a strong correlation between the prevalence of asthma and long-term exposure to allergen, and asthma often improves when the allergen is removed, although this is not always feasible.

Domestic mites appear to be the most common sources of indoor allergens. The principal species involved are *Dermatophagoides pteronyssinus*, *D. farinae*, *D. microceras* and *Euroglyphus mainei*; these account for about 90% of mites in house dust in temperate climates. The predominant allergens are amylase, and cysteine and serine proteases from the digestive tracts of the mites and their feces. In inner cities and tropical environments, cockroaches are also a source of asthmagenic allergens.

Domestic animals release allergens in their saliva, urine, feces and danders. The most important allergen is the Fel d 1 allergen found in cat fur and saliva. Allergic sensitivity to dogs is less common but, nevertheless, up to 30% of allergic patients have positive skin tests to dog allergens. Other domestic pets, particularly horses, rabbits, guinea pigs, rats, gerbils and mice, are also important sources of sensitizing allergen.

Both indoor and outdoor fungi can act as allergens. The most important indoor fungi are *Penicillium*, *Aspergillus*, *Alternaria*, *Cladosporium* and *Candida spp*. *Alternaria* and *Cladosporium spp*. are also outdoor allergens. Pollen allergens associated with asthma are derived from trees (predominantly in early spring), grasses (late spring and summer) and weeds (late summer and autumn).

Occupation-related factors are summarized in Table 1.4. High-molecular-weight sensitizers such as grain, dust, urine and dander proteins from animals probably cause sensitization by the same IgE-dependent mechanisms as allergens. The mechanism by which low-molecular-weight sensitizers such as diisocyanates and platinum salts act is unknown; however, there is increasing evidence that IgE plays a role here too.

Drugs. Among the most common causes of drug-induced asthma are acetylsalicylic acid (ASA; aspirin) and other non-steroidal anti-inflammatory drugs (NSAIDs), which trigger asthma attacks in 4–28% of asthmatic patients in different countries. Intolerance to NSAIDs usually develops between 30 and 50 years of age, and persists throughout life. It may result from a defect in the oxidative metabolism of arachidonic acid, causing excessive production of a powerful class of bronchoconstricting mediators – the cysteinyl leukotrienes (cysLTs). Individuals with ASA-intolerant asthma are commonly not atopic. They may also have nasal polyposis.

Exposure to cigarette smoke is one of the potentially modifiable causes of asthma. Passive exposure is an important early-life risk factor for asthma, impairing lung growth and encouraging allergic responses in early infancy. Children exposed to cigarette smoke, especially from their mothers, have a significantly increased risk of asthma and exacerbations. In adults, there is some evidence that smoking may increase the risk of developing asthma after exposure to some occupational sensitizers. In addition, current smoking is associated with an increase in symptoms and blunted response to preventive treatments, especially steroids.

Pollution. Laboratory studies have identified a number of air pollutants as factors in worsening asthma, but epidemiological studies of the relationship between outdoor air pollution and asthma have

TABLE 1.4

Some causes of occupational asthma

Occupation/occupational field	Agent
	Animal proteins
Laboratory animal workers, vets	Dander and urine proteins
Food processing	Shellfish, egg proteins, pancreatic enzymes, amylase
Dairy farmers	Storage mites
Poultry farmers	Poultry mites, droppings, feathers
Granary workers	Storage mites, *Aspergillus spp.*, indoor ragweed, grass
Research workers	Locusts
Fish-food manufacturing	Midges
Detergent manufacturing	*Bacillus subtilis* enzymes
Silk workers	Silkworm moths and larvae
	Plant proteins
Bakers	Flour, amylase
Food processing	Coffee-bean dust, meat tenderizer (papain), tea
Farmers	Soybean dust
Shipping workers	Grain dust (mold, insects, grain)
Laxative manufacturing	Ispaghula, psyllium
Sawmill workers, carpenters	Wood dust (western red cedar, oak, mahogany, zebrawood, redwood, Lebanon cedar, African maple, eastern white cedar)
Electric soldering	Colophony (pine resin)
Nurses	Psyllium, latex

CONTINUED

TABLE 1.4 (CONTINUED)

Occupation/occupational field	Agent
	Inorganic chemicals
Refinery workers	Platinum salts, vanadium salts
Plating	Nickel salts
Diamond polishing	Cobalt salts
Manufacturing	Aluminum fluoride
Beauticians	Persulfate
Welding	Stainless-steel fumes, chromium salts
	Organic chemicals
Manufacturing	Antibiotics, piperazine, methyldopa, salbutamol, cimetidine
Hospital workers	Disinfectants (sulfathiazole, chloramines, formaldehyde, glutaraldehyde), latex
Anesthesiology	Enflurane
Fur dyeing	Fur dye
Rubber processing	Formaldehyde, ethylene diamine, phthalic anhydride, triethylene tetramines, trimellitic anhydride, hexamethyl tetramine, acrylates
Automobile painting	Ethanolamine, diisocyanates
Foundry workers	Reaction product of furan binder

yielded conflicting results. Although asthma is more common in industrialized countries (see Chapter 2), there is little evidence that air pollution alone is directly responsible for this increase in prevalence. Importantly, indoor pollutants arising from, for example, heating and cooking with gas or on wood fires, and organic chemicals used in buildings and furnishings appear to be associated with increases in prevalence in some instances. Exposure to air pollution can also exacerbate established asthma.

Diet. The relationship between asthma and dietary factors is unclear. There is some evidence that asthma is associated with food allergy during infancy, which often precedes other atopic disorders such as allergic rhinitis and, frequently, asthma. Several trials of dietary modification to avoid highly 'allergenic' foods in pregnancy and in the first year of life have shown some benefit in delaying the onset of allergic diseases, but not in reducing the eventual occurrence of asthma. Therefore, dietary modifications during pregnancy and infancy to prevent asthma are not currently recommended. Babies should be breastfed exclusively for the first 6 months of life.

Epidemiological evidence suggests that diets high in omega-3 fatty acids (mainly acquired from fish oils) may be protective against asthma, as may diets high in antioxidants (from fruit and vegetables). However, these findings await confirmation from large prospective controlled trials.

Infections. Viral infections are well established as a cause of asthma exacerbations; they have been detected in over 80% of children with an exacerbation. The role of particular infections, such as respiratory syncytial virus, as a cause of asthma in early life is becoming increasingly well established by large cohort studies (see Chapter 2).

Obesity is considered a major risk factor for asthma. Obesity-induced changes in hormones metabolized in adipose tissue may lead to a low-grade systemic inflammation that involves the lung. In addition, some of the comorbidities of obesity, such as gastroesophageal reflux and sleep-disordered breathing, may trigger asthma or asthma-like symptoms.

Trigger factors can induce asthma by causing inflammation, provoking bronchial hyperresponsiveness or both. Individual triggers vary markedly, and may also alter with time in the same patient. Common triggers include allergens, air pollutants, viral infections, exercise and hyperventilation, and emotional stress. In addition, adverse weather conditions have been associated with asthma exacerbations.

Key points – pathophysiology

- Asthma is a chronic inflammatory condition of the conducting airways. It is characterized by recurrent episodes of airflow limitation which, depending on the severity of the attack, can cause breathlessness, wheezing, chest tightness and cough.
- Structural changes also occur; these are particularly evident in those with severe and chronic asthma.
- The most prominent risk factors are allergen exposure in genetically susceptible individuals and maternal cigarette smoking.
- Genetic factors determine susceptibility to environmental factors, and it is the interaction between these that leads to clinical disease.

Key references

Anderson GP. Endotyping asthma: new insights into key pathogenic mechanisms in a complex, heterogeneous disease. *Lancet* 2008;372:1107–19.

Arshad SH. Primary prevention of asthma and allergy. *J Allergy Clin Immunol* 2005;116:3–14.

Haldar P, Pavord ID. Noneosinophilic asthma: a distinct clinical and pathologic phenotype. *J Allergy Clin Immunol* 2007;119: 1043–52.

Holgate ST. Epithelium dysfunction in asthma. *J Allergy Clin Immunol* 2007;120:1233–44.

Holloway JW, Yang IA, Holgate ST. Interpatient variability in rates of asthma progression: can genetics provide an answer? *J Allergy Clin Immunol* 2008;121:573–9.

Schaub B, Lauener R, von Mutius E. The many faces of the hygiene hypothesis. *J Allergy Clin Immunol* 2006;117:969–77.

Shore SA. Obesity and asthma: possible mechanisms. *J Allergy Clin Immunol* 2008;121:1087–93.

Asthma is one of the most common chronic diseases worldwide, but reliable epidemiological data are hard to obtain. The reported prevalence depends on the definition of asthma used, the age and socioeconomic status of the population studied, and the study design.

Prevalence

The prevalence of asthma in populations has been estimated to approach 20% (Figures 2.1 and 2.2). The prevalence is usually higher in children than in adults, with peak prevalence approaching 25%. Although reliable data are hard to obtain, studies have consistently shown that the prevalence of asthma increased worldwide during the 1990s. However, in countries with a very high prevalence of asthma historically, such as Australia, New Zealand and the UK, the rates of asthma have stabilized or are falling.

Within a particular country, the prevalence of asthma may differ markedly between different racial or ethnic groups. In the USA, for example, asthma is more common among black African–Americans than in whites, but the difference is less pronounced in the UK. In the UK, the prevalence among Asians is lower than among whites.

Asthma appears to be more prevalent in urbanized countries; the reasons are not clear, but may include:

- exposure to airborne allergens, particularly house dust mites
- exposure to occupational allergens
- increased urbanization and thus exposure to adjuvants such as certain respiratory viruses, dietary components and pollutants
- reduced exposure to bacterial and viral infections in early infancy.

Asthma mortality

Death rates from asthma are usually reported for the under 35s as the report of an asthma-related death in this age group is relatively reliable (Figure 2.3). In older age groups the reported mortality from asthma can be inflated because of comorbidities, particularly chronic obstructive

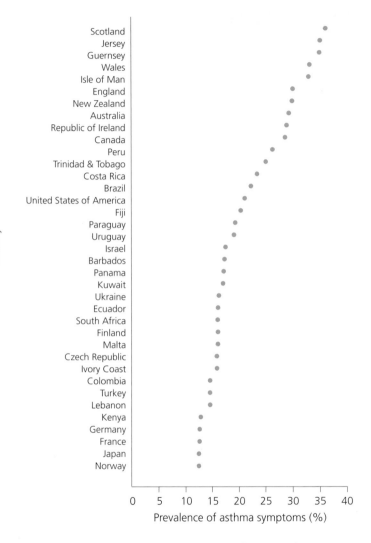

Figure 2.1 International and national variations in asthma prevalence suggest that environmental factors may affect asthma development in childhood. In the International Study of Asthma and Allergies in Childhood (ISAAC), children aged 13–14 years were asked to complete questionnaires about symptoms of asthma experienced in the past 12 months. Prevalence of self-reported wheezing ranges from 1 to 35%, with the higher prevalence rates found in more urbanized nations. Reproduced from Masoli et al. 2004, with permission from the Global Initiative for Asthma. Available at www.ginasthma.org

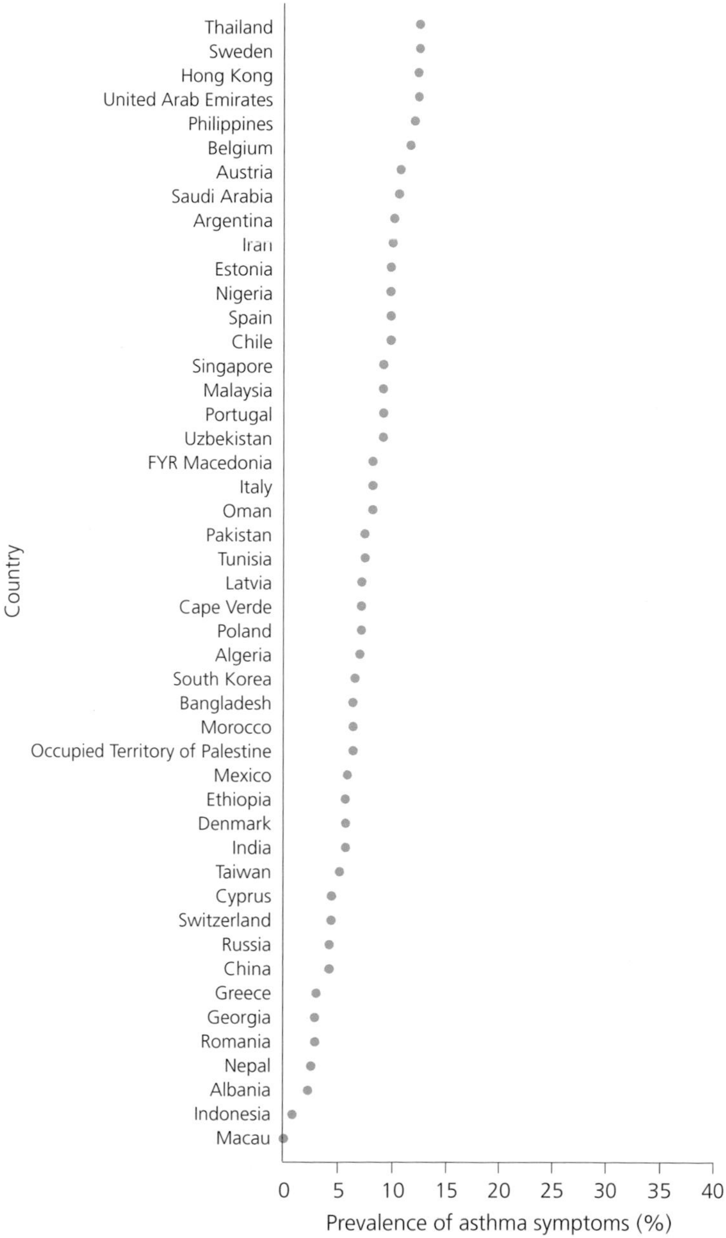

Figure 2.1 (continued)

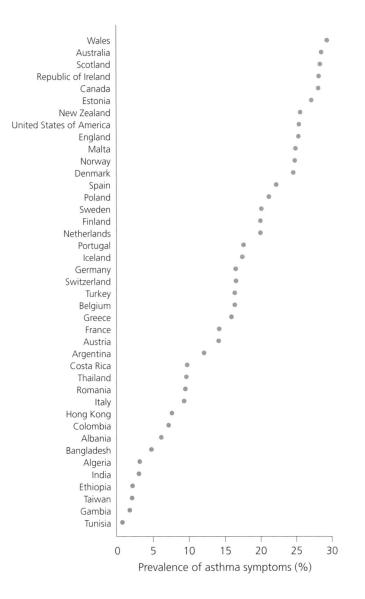

Figure 2.2 The prevalence of asthma according to questionnaire in adults aged 20 to 44 years. Prevalence rates of self-reported wheezing range from 1 to 30%. Reproduced from Masoli et al. 2004, with permission from the Global Initiative for Asthma. Available at www.ginasthma.org

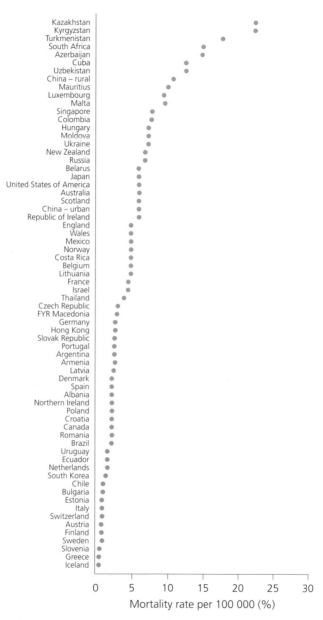

Figure 2.3 Asthma mortality in young people aged 5 to 34 years. There is substantial regional variation. Reproduced from Masoli et al. 2004, with permission from the Global Initiative for Asthma. Available at www.ginasthma.org

pulmonary disease (COPD). Mortality rates are often higher in more urbanized nations. Wide variation in case-fatality rates is seen worldwide (Figure 2.4), which may reflect differences in both the availability and the delivery of effective asthma care and medication to individuals with asthma.

Asthma death rates not only vary between nations but have also fluctuated over time. In many countries, a marked increase in asthma deaths occurred in the 1960s, after which mortality tended to decrease. In the UK, the mortality rate increased slightly during the 1980s, but the most recent data suggest that death rates are now falling. The greatest increase in mortality during the late 1970s and 1980s was seen in New Zealand (Figure 2.5). The reasons for this are unclear; the use of high doses of short-acting β_2-agonists (SABAs), especially fenoterol, has been associated with the increased mortality, but the evidence is inconclusive. Ethnic and socioeconomic factors may be at least partly responsible. In

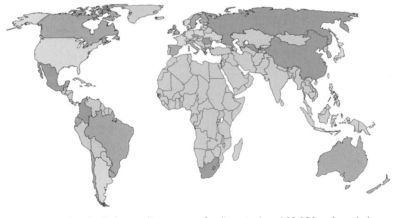

Countries shaded according to case-fatality rate (per 100 000 asthmatics)

- ■ > 10.0
- ■ 0–5.0
- ▢ 5.1–10.0
- ▢ No standardized data available

Figure 2.4 Asthma mortality rates in individual countries where data are available, adjusted for the asthma prevalence in that nation. The substantial variation suggests that access to treatment and other preventive measures are likely to influence asthma mortality rates. Reproduced from Masoli et al. 2004, with permission from the Global Initiative for Asthma. Available at

www.ginasthma.org

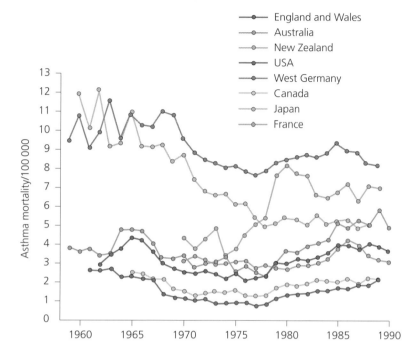

Figure 2.5 Deaths from asthma in patients of all ages, 1960–1990.

New Zealand, a large proportion of the increased mortality occurred in Maoris, and during the same period a similar increase occurred among black Americans living in inner-city areas of the USA. Studies of asthma deaths during this time suggested that a majority were preventable with the best available current treatment, and that factors such as poor access to healthcare may have been partly responsible. In countries that have introduced effective guidelines for asthma management (e.g. the UK, Australia and Scandinavian countries), mortality is now declining.

Asthma morbidity

In addition to being an important cause of death, asthma causes substantial morbidity and interference with everyday activities. Insights into the extent of asthma-related morbidity come from studies of hospital admission rates, which have shown that hospitalizations for asthma are increasing in a number of countries.

Increasing morbidity may relate to a number of factors, including:
- the increasing prevalence of asthma
- increased exposure to trigger factors (e.g. allergens, pollutants, viruses)
- undertreatment with, or reduced access to, anti-inflammatory agents
- overdependence on bronchodilators
- failure to monitor lung function by regular peak expiratory flow (PEF) measurements or spirometry
- delay in seeking medical attention during acute exacerbations.

In addition, in affluent countries, low income appears to be a risk factor for increased morbidity.

Early-life origins of asthma

Studies in neonates and young children born of allergic parents suggest that the atopic state begins to manifest itself very early in life. Thus, the findings of increased numbers of mast cells and eosinophils in the lavage fluid of children with asthma aged 3–5 years suggest that all the necessary cell and mediator pathways are already in place to express the full disease. Despite several recent large intervention studies, such as the Childhood Asthma Management Program (CAMP) and START (Inhaled Steroid Treatment As Regular Therapy In Early Asthma), it is still not clear whether the introduction of inhaled corticosteroids early in life, at the onset of asthma, influences the natural history of the disease or airway remodeling; two recent studies suggest that it does not.

There may be maternal risk factors that influence the genetic expression of allergy and asthma in the offspring. Several laboratories have now shown that lymphocytes from the cord blood of babies of allergic mothers show delayed maturation, particularly in respect of the cytokine interferon-γ, which, under normal conditions, has the capacity to inhibit the development of the allergic pathways. The basis for this deficiency is far from clear, but it does provide one potential avenue for correcting an immunologic response early in life before the allergic cells are recruited into the lung.

Natural history of asthma

Asthma can occur at any time in life, although it most commonly develops in infancy and childhood. The natural history of the condition varies according to the age at onset, and possibly according to the causative factors.

Infancy. Wheezing is common in the early years of life and recent studies have enabled the identification of several distinct phenotypes. The most common are:

- transient infantile wheeze, in which children have recurrent wheeze during the first few years of life, but rarely thereafter
- episodic wheeze, where children have wheeze associated with viral infections that does not persist between attacks
- atopic asthma, in which children are usually allergic and often have other allergic diseases such as allergic rhinitis and eczema.

Atopic asthma is generally more likely to persist into childhood than the other wheezing phenotypes, whilst episodic wheezing may resolve later in childhood.

Childhood. Allergy, particularly to house-dust mites, is the most common feature associated with the development of asthma during childhood. Viral infections are important triggers of exacerbations in children with atopic asthma, but there is little evidence that they are a direct cause of asthma development. By the age of 8 years, a significant proportion of children develop bronchial hyperresponsiveness and symptoms of moderate-to-severe asthma, whereas others continue to show mild intermittent asthma.

Lung growth is relatively normal in most children with mild asthma, but may be reduced in children with severe persistent symptoms. This is important – long-term studies show that, although asthma disappears in 30–50% of children during puberty, it often recurs in adulthood. Furthermore, lung function often remains impaired even when clinical signs of asthma have disappeared, and 5–10% of children with mild asthma develop severe asthma later in life. In general, children with mild asthma are likely to have a good prognosis, but those with moderate or severe asthma are likely to show some degree of bronchial hyperresponsiveness and to be at risk of the persistence of asthma throughout life.

There is no evidence that regular use of corticosteroids in early life alters the natural history of asthma, though these drugs are highly effective in disease control. There is evidence that eczema is a major risk for the persistence of childhood asthma into adult life.

Prevalence studies reveal that asthma is generally more common in boys until puberty, when more girls develop asthma and the predominance reverses. Many individuals acquire asthma in their adolescent years.

Adulthood. The development of asthma in adulthood is frequently associated with exposure to occupational sensitizers causing classic allergic responses or via mechanisms not involving immunoglobulin E. It is not known what proportion of patients who develop asthma in adulthood actually had a history of childhood asthma; abnormal lung

---

Key points – epidemiology and natural history

- Asthma is one of the most common chronic diseases worldwide. The highest prevalence is seen in affluent westernized populations.
- In many countries asthma, along with other allergic disorders, continues to increase in prevalence, especially in children and young adults.
- Death from asthma reflects poor access to healthcare in many countries.
- Asthma can occur at any time in life, although it most commonly develops in infancy and childhood.
- There is evidence that early life events, including those that occur in the womb, may be important in the initiation of childhood asthma in those genetically at risk.
- Although asthma disappears in 30–50% of children during puberty, it often recurs in adulthood.
- There is no evidence that regular use of corticosteroids in early life alters the natural history of asthma, though these medications are highly effective in disease control.

function or bronchial hyperresponsiveness persists in many patients whose symptoms disappear during childhood.

The natural history of late-onset asthma is variable. It appears that lung function (as measured by the forced expiratory volume in 1 second [FEV_1]) deteriorates at a faster rate in patients whose asthma develops after the age of about 50 years than in those who develop asthma at an earlier age. Moreover, bronchial hyperresponsiveness appears to be associated with a faster rate of deterioration. Such older people with asthma have increasingly become the focus of attention as the mortality of this group is relatively high.

Key references

Asher MI, Montefort S, Björkstén B et al. Worldwide time trends in the prevalence of symptoms of asthma, allergic rhinoconjunctivitis, and eczema in childhood: ISAAC Phases One and Three repeat multicountry cross-sectional surveys. *Lancet* 2006;368:733–43.

The Childhood Asthma Management Program Research Group. Long-term effects of budesonide or nedocromil in children with asthma. *N Engl J Med* 2000;343:1054–63.

Holt PG, Upham JW, Sly PD. Contemporaneous maturation of immunologic and respiratory functions during early childhood: implications for development of asthma prevention strategies. *J Allergy Clin Immunol* 2005; 116:16–24.

Lowe AJ, Carlin JB, Bennett CM et al. Do boys do the atopic march while girls dawdle? *J Allergy Clin Immunol* 2008;121:1190–5.

Masoli M, Fabian D, Holt S, Beasley R. *Global Burden of Asthma*. Report developed for the Global Initiative for Asthma, 2004. www.ginasthma.org

Pauwels RA, Pedersen S, Busse WW et al. Early intervention with budesonide in mild persistent asthma: a randomised, double-blind trial. *Lancet* 2003;361:1071–6.

Sly PD, Boner AL, Björksten B et al. Early identification of atopy in the prediction of persistent asthma in children. *Lancet* 2008;372:1100–6.

3 Diagnosis and classification

Although asthma is one of the most common chronic disorders it is often underdiagnosed, especially in older people. Because of the intermittent and non-specific nature of symptoms, patients may accept the effects of their condition and delay seeking treatment. They may also be incorrectly diagnosed when they do seek medical advice: asthma is often misdiagnosed as bronchitis or 'wheezy' bronchitis, particularly in children and the elderly, and is treated inappropriately with antibiotics. An accurate diagnosis is essential for effective asthma control.

Symptoms

The clinical diagnosis of asthma is often based on the presence of symptoms such as:

- breathlessness – often episodic
- wheezing
- chest tightness
- coughing.

These symptoms may be particularly marked at night and in the early hours of the morning.

The presence of symptoms, however, is not by itself sufficient for a diagnosis of asthma; the history of symptoms and possible provocative factors must also be considered (Table 3.1), and the diagnosis confirmed by objective measures of lung function.

Various symptom scoring scales have been developed to monitor the occurrence and severity of symptoms. These can be useful in the management of individual patients, although it is important that they be adapted according to the patient's age and cultural background.

Physical examination

Asthma symptoms vary during the day, and the respiratory system may appear normal on physical examination. During asthma exacerbations, small airways are occluded through a combination of bronchoconstriction, edema and hypersecretion of mucus. The patient

TABLE 3.1

Key questions to consider in making a diagnosis of asthma

Consider asthma if the answer to any of the following is 'yes'

- Has the patient had an attack or recurrent episodes of wheezing?
- Does the patient have a troublesome cough, particularly at night or on waking?
- Is the patient awoken by coughing or difficulty in breathing?
- Does the patient cough or wheeze after physical activity?
- Does the patient experience breathing difficulties during a particular season?
- Does the patient cough, wheeze or develop chest tightness after exposure to airborne allergens or irritants?
- Do colds go to the chest or take more than 10 days to resolve?
- Does the patient use any medication when symptoms occur? If so, how often?
- Are symptoms relieved when medication is used?

therefore breathes at a higher lung volume to maintain airway patency. Consequently, clinical signs of dyspnea (Table 3.2) are more likely to be present during symptomatic exacerbations or if patients are examined in the morning before administration of a bronchodilator.

The absence of wheezing is not sufficient to preclude a diagnosis of asthma. In an exacerbation, some patients may have such severe obstruction of the airways that wheezing may not be noticeable. Such patients usually have other signs of respiratory obstruction, such as difficulty in speaking, cyanosis, drowsiness and chest hyperinflation.

Measurements of lung function

Patients with asthma often have poor recognition of their symptoms and poor perception of symptom severity. Measurements of lung function provide an objective assessment of airflow limitation, and its variability and reversibility, and thus are valuable in the diagnosis and management of asthma. Measurements widely used in patients over 5 years of age are

TABLE 3.2

Clinical signs of asthma

- Dyspnea
  - wheezing, particularly on expiration
  - use of the accessory muscles of respiration
  - flaring of the nostrils during inspiration (particularly in children)
  - interrupted talking
  - hyperinflation (use of accessory muscles, hunched shoulders, hunching forward or preferring not to lie down)
- Cough
  - chronic or recurring
  - worse at night and in the early hours of the morning; sleep disrupted
- Tachycardia
- Associated conditions
  - eczema
  - rhinitis
  - sinusitis
  - hay fever
- Cyanosis – life-threatening!
- Drowsiness – life-threatening!

forced expiratory volume in 1 second (FEV_1), forced vital capacity (FVC) and peak expiratory flow (PEF).

FEV_1 and FVC are measured by spirometry. To make these measurements, patients are taught to perform a forced expiration after a maximal inspiration, and the highest of at least three reproducible measurements is recorded. Predicted values based on age, sex, race and height are available and can be compared with the patient's measurements to aid interpretation. The ratio of FEV_1 to FVC provides a useful measure of airway obstruction. Forced expiration normally produces FEV_1/FVC ratios of more than 70% (or 85% in children); ratios below these figures suggest airway obstruction: the lower the ratio, the more severe the obstruction.

Spirometers have become smaller and more portable; while spirometry is usually carried out in the hospital or specialist setting, it is increasingly available in an office setting, such as a general practice room. If spirometry is used to monitor patients, it is critical that the tester is appropriately trained in conducting the test and in maintaining the equipment to ensure reproducibility and comparability of measurements. For asthma diagnosis, spirometry is usually assessed before and after the administration of an inhaled short-acting β_2-agonist (SABA): responsiveness of FEV_1 by 15% or 200 mL (whichever is the greater) is indicative of asthma.

Measurement of PEF by means of a peak flow meter provides a useful and practical alternative to spirometry. In most patients, there is a good correlation between PEF and FEV_1.

Peak flow meters are small, convenient, inexpensive and suitable for home use. They can therefore be used both for the diagnosis of asthma in the clinic (Table 3.3) and to monitor asthma in the home. Changes in PEF can precede the onset of symptoms during acute exacerbations in some individuals; thus, early detection of such changes can allow appropriate treatment to be given. PEF readings can also indicate to an individual the severity of their asthma when compared with previous readings, enabling institution of a self-management plan.

Several types of peak flow meter are available, but the basic technique for use is the same in each case (Figure 3.1). Ideally, patients

TABLE 3.3

Diagnosis of asthma from peak expiratory flow (PEF) measurements

- PEF increases by more than 15% and at least 60 L/min 15–20 minutes after inhalation of a short-acting β_2-agonist (e.g. salbutamol or terbutaline)

- PEF varies by more than 20% between morning measurement on waking and measurement 12 hours later

- PEF decreases by more than 15% after 6 minutes of running or other exercise

Put the disposable mouthpiece on the peak flow meter.

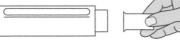
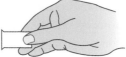

Stand up and hold the peak flow meter horizontally. Make sure that the end of the marker is at the end of the scale and that your hand is not restricting marker movement.

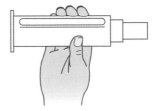

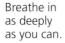

Breathe in as deeply as you can.

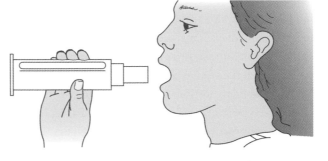

Then close your lips tightly around the mouthpiece and breathe out quickly. Note the results and repeat the procedure twice. Use the highest reading.

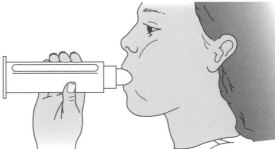

Figure 3.1 Use of a peak flow meter.

should measure PEF immediately on waking before taking any bronchodilator medication and last thing at night after taking bronchodilator. Variability in daily PEF can then be calculated as a percentage of the mean daily value:

$$\text{Daily variability (\%)} = \frac{\text{PEF}_{evening} - \text{PEF}_{morning}}{{}^{1}/_{2}\,(\text{PEF}_{evening} + \text{PEF}_{morning})} \times 100$$

Daily variability of more than 20% indicates asthma.

Measurement of bronchial responsiveness

Measurement of bronchial responsiveness can be useful in the diagnosis of asthma, although there is some overlap between the range of values found in patients with asthma and in those with rhinitis or other causes of lower airway obstruction, such as chronic obstructive pulmonary disease (COPD). The most usual tests are performed in a lung function laboratory and involve the patient inhaling incremental doses of a bronchoconstricting substance, such as histamine, methacholine, hypertonic saline, adenosine 5'-monophosphate (AMP) or mannitol. Spirometry is then used to follow the changes in airway caliber. Airway responsiveness is usually defined as that dose (D) or concentration (C) of agonist that reduces the FEV_1 by 20% of the starting volume (i.e. PD_{20} or PC_{20}). A standardized exercise test is also useful, especially for children with suspected asthma.

Skin-prick tests

Skin-prick tests with allergens or detection of allergen-specific immunoglobulin (Ig)E in the circulation are the most common diagnostic tests for allergy. For the diagnosis of asthma, the results should always be interpreted in relation to the patient's history and the relationship between asthma symptoms and allergen exposure, because up to 40% of the population may exhibit atopy but only a proportion of these individuals will have asthma. Nevertheless, the identification of allergens that may be contributing to persistent asthma and exacerbations is important in order to provide advice on allergen avoidance or other treatment strategies.

Patient groups

The diagnosis of asthma may be difficult in certain patient groups, especially smokers and the extremely young or old, who may have difficulty performing lung function tests.

Infants may have recurrent wheezing due to acute viral respiratory infections; the first episode of wheezing in infants under 6 months of age is usually due to viral bronchiolitis, whereas asthma is more likely to be the cause of wheezing after 18 months of age. After a viral infection, symptoms may persist in children with atopic asthma. Similarly, older children may show asthma symptoms in association with viral infections or exercise; asthma should be considered if the child has a persistent nocturnal cough, or if colds go to the chest easily or take longer than 10 days to resolve.

Elderly patients. In older people, asthma may coexist with conditions such as COPD, bronchiectasis or interstitial pulmonary fibrosis. A history of asthma in childhood and variability on spirometry or PEF testing with β_2-agonists supports the diagnosis.

Occupational asthma is often misdiagnosed as chronic bronchitis or COPD. Ideally, diagnosis requires a detailed occupational history and the demonstration of a clear relationship between the development of symptoms at work and resolution of symptoms away from work.

Seasonal asthma associated with aero-allergens, such as the allergic rhinitis ('hay fever') suffered in the spring by pollen-sensitive individuals, may present as intermittent symptoms, with the patient being asymptomatic between seasons, or as seasonal worsening of moderate or severe asthma.

Cough-variant asthma. Patients present with cough as the principal symptom; they seldom wheeze. Coughing is often confined to the night, and examination during the day may not reveal evidence of abnormalities. Lung function tests and measurement of bronchial responsiveness with some form of challenge test are particularly important in these patients. Another helpful sign is eosinophils in the sputum (eosinophilic bronchitis).

Differential diagnosis

Wheezing can arise from either widespread or localized airway obstruction, and this should be considered in the differential diagnosis (Figure 3.2).

Breathlessness and cough are common symptoms of many conditions. The keys to diagnosing asthma are the patient's history together with measurements of lung function through spirometry. An obstructive ventilatory defect suggests asthma or COPD while excluding other conditions. In adults, asthma-like symptoms can result from bronchitis or COPD; concomitant asthma and COPD are common among past or present smokers, and even occur in some individuals who have never smoked. Demonstration of reversible and variable airflow limitation confirms the diagnosis of asthma and indicates a trial of preventive treatment.

Although it is not always possible to distinguish asthma and COPD in those with a fixed component of airflow obstruction, detection of

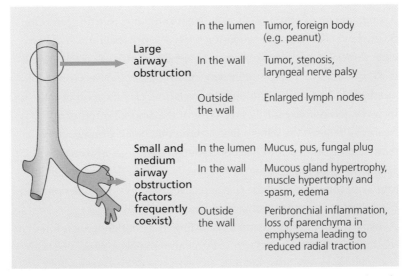

Figure 3.2 Differential diagnosis of obstructive airway disease. Reproduced with permission from Professor Martyn R Partridge, Imperial College London.

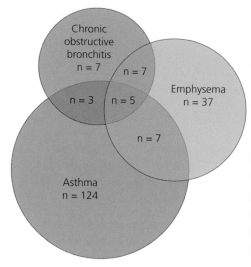

Figure 3.3 The distribution of obstructive airways disease in a middle-aged population. While COPD and emphysema are present, reversible airflow obstruction (asthma) was the most common cause of airflow obstruction in this group of patients. Reproduced with permission from Abramson M. *MJA* 2005;183(1 suppl): S23–5.

airflow obstruction warrants a trial of therapy with inhaled corticosteroids to assess reversibility and asthma still appears to be the most likely diagnosis in middle-aged adults (Figure 3.3).

Classification of asthma severity

A combination of symptom measurements and lung function tests can be used to classify asthma according to its severity (Figure 3.4). These clinical measures of disease severity have been shown to correlate well with pathological markers of airway inflammation such as eosinophil numbers. Despite this pathological correlation, classification of asthma by severity is not necessarily predictive of the amount or types of treatment required to achieve best asthma outcomes. Consequently, treatment algorithms are based on asthma control: an assessment of symptoms including daytime symptoms, limitation of activities, night-time symptoms, the need for rescue reliever therapy, lung function, and exacerbation frequency and severity (see Chapter 4).

Asthma can also be classified according to the inflammation found in the airways. Whilst characteristically asthma has been associated with eosinophilic airway inflammation, the presence of non-eosinophilic inflammation may suggest types of asthma that are more likely to be relatively corticosteroid resistant. Non-invasive assessment of airway

Step 4: severe persistent

- Symptoms daily
- Frequent exacerbations
- Frequent nocturnal asthma symptoms
- Limitation of physical activities
- FEV_1 or PEF ≤ 60% predicted
- PEF or FEV_1 variability > 30%

Step 3: moderate persistent

- Symptoms daily
- Exacerbations may affect activity and sleep
- Nocturnal symptoms more than once a week
- Daily use of inhaled short-acting β_2-agonist
- FEV_1 or PEF 60–80% predicted
- PEF or FEV_1 variability > 30%

Step 2: mild persistent

- Symptoms more than once a week but less than once a day
- Exacerbations may affect activity and sleep
- Nocturnal symptoms more than twice a month
- FEV_1 or PEF ≥ 80% predicted
- PEF or FEV_1 variability < 20–30%

Step 1: intermittent

- Symptoms less than once a week
- Brief exacerbations
- Nocturnal symptoms not more than twice a month
- FEV_1 or PEF ≥ 80% predicted
- PEF or FEV_1 variability < 20%

Figure 3.4 Classification of asthma severity by clinical features (before treatment). The worst feature determines the classification of severity. FEV_1, forced expiratory volume in 1 second; PEF, peak expiratory flow. From Global Initiative for Asthma, 2008. www.ginasthma.org

inflammation can be performed by analysing induced sputum for cellular types. The analysis of sputum inflammatory cells has been used to guide asthma treatment, some reports finding that this mode of therapy may be effective in preventing asthma exacerbations. The measurement of the concentration of nitric oxide in exhaled air can be used as a surrogate measure for airway inflammation, though this measurement is very sensitive to corticosteroid therapy.

In assessing the severity of illness it is important to remember that patients often have a poor perception of the potential severity of their asthma, largely because they have adapted their lifestyle to accommodate their disease. There is also often a lack of lung function measurements to provide more objective information. It is important to recognize that even mild asthma can be associated with severe, potentially fatal exacerbations. Risk factors that have been shown to be associated with an increased risk of death from asthma include:

- a previous history of acute life-threatening attacks
- hospitalization for asthma within the previous year
- psychosocial problems
- a history of intubation for asthma
- recent reduction or cessation of systemic corticosteroid therapy
- non-adherence to preventive treatments
- difficulty accessing treatment.

Conversely, a written asthma action plan has been found to be protective against asthma death.

Key points – diagnosis and classification

- Although asthma is one of the most common chronic disorders, it is often underdiagnosed.
- The clinical diagnosis of asthma is often based on the presence of symptoms, such as breathlessness (often episodic), wheezing, chest tightness and coughing.
- Objective measures of lung function are important in order to establish asthma as a diagnosis and to assess the response to treatment.
- Measurement of bronchial responsiveness and allergy status can aid diagnosis as well as identify possible preventive measures.
- Attempts should be made to assess disease control to guide treatment.
- The diagnosis of asthma may be difficult in certain patient groups, especially those who smoke and the very young or old.

Key references

Chen H, Gould MK, Blanc PD et al. Asthma control, severity and quality of life: quantifying the effect of uncontrolled disease. *J Allergy Clin Immunol* 2007;120:396–402.

Global Initiative for Asthma. *Global Strategy for Asthma Management and Prevention*, Updated 2008. Available at www.ginasthma.org

Haldar P, Pavord ID. Noneosinophilic asthma: a distinct clinical and pathologic phenotype. *J Allergy Clin Immunol* 2007;119:1043–52.

Johns DP, Pierce R. *Pocket Guide to Spirometry*, 2nd edn. Sydney: McGraw-Hill, 2007.

The aims of asthma management are summarized in Table 4.1. Successful achievement of these aims requires attention to preventive measures such as allergen avoidance (see Chapter 6), and the use of medication to prevent symptoms from developing and to treat acute attacks. Drugs used in the management of asthma can be classified as controllers (also called preventers) and relievers.

Controller (preventer) medications

Controllers (preventers) are taken daily over the long term to control persistent asthma (Table 4.2). They include anti-inflammatory agents such as corticosteroids, sodium cromoglicate, nedocromil sodium and leukotriene modifiers, and long-acting bronchodilators such as long-acting β_2-agonists (LABAs) and sustained-release theophylline.

Inhaled corticosteroids, such as beclometasone (beclomethasone) dipropionate, budesonide, fluticasone propionate, mometasone, fluticasone furoate and ciclesonide, are the most effective anti-inflammatory agents currently available for asthma management. Studies have consistently shown that these agents reduce pathological signs of airway inflammation, so that lung function and symptoms improve, bronchial hyperresponsiveness decreases, and the frequency

TABLE 4.1

Aims of asthma management

- Control symptoms
- Prevent exacerbations
- Maintain pulmonary function as close to normal levels as possible
- Maintain normal levels of activity
- Prevent the development of irreversible airflow limitation
- Prevent asthma mortality

TABLE 4.2

Effects of anti-asthma drugs and risks of serious adverse events during long-term use

	Control of symptoms over weeks to months	Relief of exacerbations over minutes or hours	Risk of serious long-term adverse events
Inhaled corticosteroids	+++	–	+ (at high doses)
Oral corticosteroids (prednisolone)	++	++ (over hours)	+++
Sodium cromoglicate	+	–	–
Nedocromil sodium	+	–	–
Leukotriene modifiers	++	+	–
Short-acting inhaled β_2-agonists	+/–	+++	–
Long-acting inhaled β_2-agonists	++	++/+++	–
Oral β_2-agonists	+/–	+	+
Theophylline	+	++	++
Omalizumab	++	–	+
Inhaled anticholinergic agents	+	++	–

and severity of exacerbations are reduced. Corticosteroids interrupt the signaling pathways for pro-inflammatory molecules by decreasing the expression of genes for a variety of inflammatory mediators and by increasing the expression of genes for anti-inflammatory mediators.

Inhaled corticosteroids are also useful in the treatment of severe persistent asthma because they reduce the need for oral corticosteroids and have fewer systemic adverse effects. Local adverse effects, which include oropharyngeal candidiasis, dysphonia and coughing, can largely be prevented by using spacer devices and mouth rinsing after use. Potential systemic adverse effects include thinning of the skin, cataract formation, adrenal suppression and decreased bone metabolism and growth. The risk of such effects depends on a number of factors, including the dose taken, absorption from the gut or lung, the extent of first-pass metabolism in the gut wall and liver, and the half-life of the corticosteroid. In general, the risk of significant systemic effects is low with therapeutic doses.

Systemic corticosteroids, such as prednisolone, can be given either orally or parenterally. Short courses (5–7 days) can be used when starting therapy in patients with uncontrolled asthma or during periods of worsening asthma. Long-term treatment may be necessary in patients with severe persistent asthma; patients who require such medication should be seen by a specialist. Systemic events associated with oral corticosteroids include impairment of growth in children, osteoporosis, arterial hypertension, adrenal suppression, obesity, thinning of the skin, muscle weakness, cataract formation and diabetes. It should be noted that the safety of long-term inhaled corticosteroid therapy is better than that of oral or parenteral therapy.

Leukotriene modifiers. The cysteinyl leukotrienes (cysLTs) – LTC_4, LTD_4 and LTE_4 – are potent mediators of asthma. They are generated from arachidonic acid by the 5-lipoxygenase pathway that operates in mast cells and eosinophils. Once known as 'slow-reacting substance of anaphylaxis', cysLTs released during the inflammatory process cause prolonged contraction of smooth muscle, microvascular leaking and sputum secretion, and attract eosinophils. Since the structure of the leukotrienes was elucidated in 1979, a number of leukotriene-modifying drugs have been developed and introduced into the market. Zafirlukast, montelukast and pranlukast are anti-asthma drugs that inhibit the effect of leukotrienes at their receptor (cysteinyl leukotriene receptor, cysLTR1). In addition, inhibitors of 5-lipoxygenase, such as zileuton, interrupt the conversion of arachidonic acid into leukotrienes, including the cysLTs and leukotriene B_4.

Treatment with one of these oral drugs can produce improvement in pulmonary function, protection from exercise-induced asthma and reduced eosinophilic inflammation. A clinical response is usually seen within 3 weeks of therapy, though not all patients benefit. Patients with asthma associated with intolerance to acetylsalicylic acid (ASA; aspirin) and other non-steroidal anti-inflammatory drugs (NSAIDs) seem to be particularly responsive.

Leukotriene modifiers can be used to treat mild persistent asthma, especially in children for whom the use of inhaled corticosteroids is limited because of concerns regarding the effects on growth. However, these drugs are less effective overall than a low dose of inhaled corticosteroid. They can also be used together with an inhaled corticosteroid in moderate and severe asthma, but are less effective than the combination of an inhaled corticosteroid and an inhaled LABA. Clearly, the advantages of these drugs over other long-term controllers (preventers) are that they are orally administered and are not corticosteroids; patient acceptability and adherence is therefore likely to be good.

Sodium cromoglicate and nedocromil sodium. Inhaled sodium cromoglicate and nedocromil sodium inhibit allergen-induced airflow limitation and acute airflow limitation after exercise or exposure to cold air or sulfur dioxide. Each agent can be used as long-term therapy early in the course of asthma; a course of 4–6 weeks may be needed to determine effectiveness in a given patient. Adverse effects are few, though coughing may result from inhalation of the powder formulation. The mechanisms of action are not fully understood; they may involve a combination of inhibition of immunoglobulin (Ig)E-dependent mediator release and blockade of sensory nerve pathways. Both agents can be used as maintenance therapy for asthma but are less effective than a low dose of inhaled corticosteroids.

Sustained-release theophylline. Theophylline is a bronchodilator, and there is some evidence that it may also have anti-inflammatory effects. It is both an inhibitor of cyclic adenosine 5'-monophosphate (cAMP) phosphodiesterase and an antagonist of adenosine receptors. During long-term treatment, sustained-release theophylline controls symptoms and improves lung function. Because of its long duration of action, it is useful in controlling nocturnal symptoms that persist despite regular

TABLE 4.3

Adverse effects associated with theophylline

- Nausea
- Vomiting
- Gastrointestinal disturbances
- Tachycardia
- Palpitations

- Arrhythmias
- Headache
- Insomnia
- Convulsions

anti-inflammatory treatment. However, theophylline has a number of potentially serious adverse effects (Table 4.3); theophylline intoxication can result in seizures and death. Furthermore, the drug has a relatively narrow therapeutic index; serum concentrations producing adverse effects are close to those required for therapeutic efficacy. Appropriate dosing and monitoring are therefore essential; in general, dosing should produce a steady-state serum theophylline concentration of 5–15 µg/mL. Monitoring is advisable when treatment is started and at regular intervals thereafter. In addition, serum drug concentrations should be monitored if:

- adverse events occur with the usual dose
- the expected therapeutic benefit is not achieved
- the patient has a condition that is likely to affect theophylline metabolism (e.g. febrile illness, pregnancy, liver disease, congestive heart failure)
- the patient is receiving concomitant treatment with drugs that interact with theophylline (e.g. cimetidine, some quinolone antibiotics).

Long-acting β_2-agonists such as salmeterol and formoterol, have a duration of action of more than 12 hours. They act by relaxing airway smooth muscle, enhancing mucociliary clearance and decreasing vascular permeability; in addition, they may modulate mediator release from mast cells and basophils. Long-term treatment with inhaled preparations improves symptoms and lung function, relieves nocturnal asthma and reduces the need for short-acting β_2-agonists (SABAs). Such preparations can be used as a more effective alternative to increasing the corticosteroid dose in patients for whom standard starting doses of inhaled corticosteroids do not control symptoms. A LABA should not be given without an inhaled corticosteroid as studies have suggested this to be associated with an increase in mortality. Adverse events associated with LABAs include cardiovascular stimulation, anxiety, heartburn and tremor.

Combination therapy. A series of clinical trials has shown that the inhaled LABAs salmeterol and formoterol, when administered to patients who are already taking inhaled corticosteroids but whose asthma is poorly controlled, may produce greater improvements in pulmonary function and symptom control than would be obtained by doubling the dose of inhaled corticosteroid. Combinations of a LABA and an inhaled corticosteroid are now available in single inhalers. It would seem, therefore, that the dose–response curve for topical corticosteroids is not linear, and that the overall benefits obtained with doses of up to approximately 800 µg beclometasone dipropionate per day are as great as those that can be achieved with further increments. One possible explanation for these observations is that topical corticosteroids are able to control the inflammatory response by inhibiting cytokine and other relevant pathways. They are not able to alter, at least in the short and medium term, the behavior of the remodeled airway with its increased smooth muscle, microvasculature and thickened airway walls. In this situation, drugs that act on the airway smooth muscle and microvasculature to restore airway physiology to normal are likely to be effective.

Omalizumab is a humanized monoclonal anti-IgE antibody, which is administered every 2–4 weeks by subcutaneous injection. The dose is titrated according to patient size and the serum level of total IgE. It binds to the part of the IgE molecule that attaches to the high-affinity and low-affinity receptors on mediator-secreting cells, thereby depriving the cells of the necessary allergen-specific IgE required to trigger secretion of mediators. The net result is that the serum level of free IgE drops steeply with the first injection and then gradually, over several weeks, IgE in the airways also falls in parallel with the downregulation of IgE receptors. Generally, an effect is observed after 4–6 months of treatment with attenuation of both early- and late-phase allergen-induced bronchoconstriction in parallel with a reduction in airway inflammation, including a decrease in airway eosinophils.

Clinical trials have revealed that this anti-allergy treatment is effective in treating allergic asthma. The availability of omalizumab is limited by its expense, but the drug is considered cost-effective in the management of severe and chronic asthma, particularly in reducing exacerbations and hospitalizations. Currently, omalizumab is listed as appropriate for Step 5 asthma treatment (from GINA guidelines, see Figure 4.5): that is, for patients who have poorly controlled asthma despite maximal doses of inhaled corticosteroids and LABAs. The major side effect of this drug has been the uncommon occurrence of anaphylaxis and severe asthma episodes following administration, which can occur several hours after the injection. Consequently, most treatment guidelines recommend observing the patient for 1–2 hours after administration and provision of an anaphylaxis plan and an epinephrine (adrenaline) auto-injector for patients to take home with them.

Reliever medications

Relievers (sometimes referred to as rescue medication) are used to rapidly reverse the bronchoconstriction and associated symptoms during acute attacks (see Table 4.2). They include SABAs, LABAs with a rapid onset of action, short-acting theophylline and short-acting anticholinergic agents. The most effective forms are those that are delivered by inhalation directly to the airways.

Short-acting β_2-agonists. Inhaled SABAs, such as salbutamol and terbutaline, are used to control bronchoconstriction, and are the treatment of choice for the management of acute exacerbations and the prophylaxis of exercise-induced asthma. Oral preparations are also available and may be suitable for patients who are unable to use inhaled medication. In general, oral administration is less desirable than inhaled administration because systemic side effects such as tachycardia are more pronounced when the drug is delivered orally.

Concern has been expressed over the long-term safety of repeatedly inhaling short-acting β_2-bronchodilators. Several points are worth making in relation to the use of these quick relievers. They are certainly the best drugs for relieving acute bronchospasm, but their increased use by a patient is a sign of worsening asthma and the need for greater use of controller (preventer) drugs. The use of one canister of a metered-dose inhaler per month should certainly sound alarm bells. Regular use of SABAs is not recommended, as a refractory response may develop, and it has been suggested that asthma may worsen. In addition, it is now known that genetic β_2-adrenoceptor polymorphisms dictate the effectiveness of these drugs, particularly with regard to tachyphylaxis or the development of refractoriness; therefore SABAs should only be used for quick relief on an 'as-required' basis.

Long-acting β_2-agonists with a rapid onset of action (e.g. formoterol) can be used as bronchodilators to treat acute asthma symptoms. Because of the concerns regarding the use of a LABA without an inhaled corticosteroid, this form of therapy is usually provided in an inhaler combined with an inhaled corticosteroid. Currently, the only single inhaler approach to demonstrate effective regular preventer and as-needed reliever therapy in clincal studies is the budesonide/ formoterol combination inhaler, which provides the patient with just one type of inhaler treatment overall for their asthma. It is important to note, that not all LABAs are suitable for this form of treatment: for example, salmeterol, but not formoterol, has a delayed onset of action compared with that of short-acting bronchodilators.

Systemic corticosteroids. Oral corticosteroid preparations have a relatively slow onset of action (4–6 hours), but are extremely useful in the treatment of severe acute exacerbations because they prevent progression of the exacerbation. As a result, they also reduce the need for emergency treatment or hospitalization, prevent early relapse and reduce the morbidity associated with exacerbations. Treatment is normally continued for 3–10 days after the exacerbation; the dose can be reduced and stopped as symptoms resolve and lung function returns to the personal best level.

Anticholinergic agents. Inhaled anticholinergic agents such as ipratropium bromide or oxitropium bromide cause bronchodilatation by inhibiting postganglionic efferent vagal fibers, thereby reducing the vagal tone of the airways. They also inhibit reflex bronchoconstriction provoked by inhaled irritants. They are less effective than inhaled β_2-agonists and have a slower onset of action, taking 30–60 minutes to reach their maximum effect. They are particularly useful in acute severe asthma exacerbations and as long-term therapy for patients with chronic obstructive pulmonary disease (COPD). Adverse effects include dry mouth and a bad taste.

Short-acting theophylline. Oral treatment with short-acting theophylline has been used for pretreatment of exercise-induced asthma and for symptomatic relief. The role of theophylline in the treatment of exacerbations is controversial and, because of the high risk of adverse effects and the slow onset of action, it is now rarely used in developed countries except for acute severe life-threatening asthma.

Delivery of inhaled medication

Inhalation of aerosols or powders achieves high drug concentrations in the airways and reduces the risk of systemic adverse effects. A variety of delivery devices are available (Table 4.4). Whichever device is chosen, its use should be explained carefully to the patient (Figures 4.1 and 4.2), and the patient's technique checked regularly.

TABLE 4.4

Devices for delivery of aerosolized medication in asthma

- Pressurized metered-dose inhalers (pMDIs)
- Breath-actuated pMDIs (e.g. Autohaler)
- Dry-powder inhalers (e.g. Accuhaler, Diskhaler, Rotahaler, Spinhaler, Turbohaler*)
- Spacer devices (e.g. AeroChamber, Babyhaler, Nebuhaler, Volumatic)
- Nebulizers

*Turbuhaler in some countries.

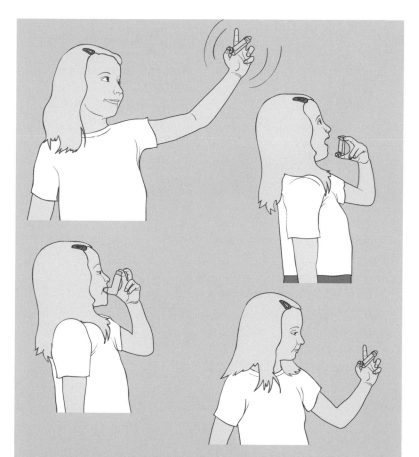

- Remove the cap from the inhaler and shake
- Breathe out gently
- Put the mouthpiece between the teeth and close lips around the mouthpiece to form a good seal
- Start to breathe in slowly through the mouth and press to actuate the puffer; continue to breathe in slowly and deeply
- Hold breath for up to 10 seconds or for as long as is comfortable
- While holding breath, remove the inhaler from mouth
- Breathe out gently
- If an extra dose is needed, wait 1 minute before repeating; replace cap

Figure 4.1 Technique for use of a metered-dose inhaler without a spacer device.

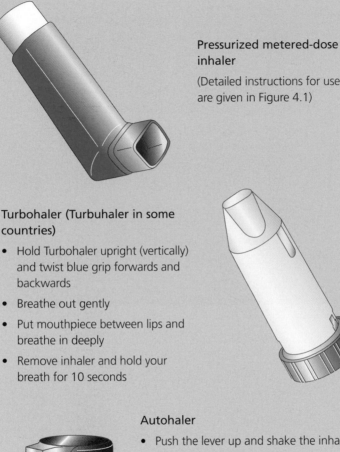

Pressurized metered-dose inhaler

(Detailed instructions for use are given in Figure 4.1)

Turbohaler (Turbuhaler in some countries)

- Hold Turbohaler upright (vertically) and twist blue grip forwards and backwards
- Breathe out gently
- Put mouthpiece between lips and breathe in deeply
- Remove inhaler and hold your breath for 10 seconds

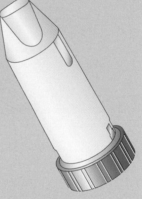

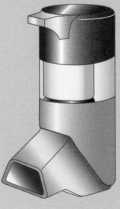

Autohaler

- Push the lever up and shake the inhaler
- Breathe out gently
- Put mouthpiece in mouth; ensure that the air vents at the bottom of the inhaler are not blocked
- Breathe in steadily; continue after the inhaler clicks
- Hold your breath for 10 seconds
- Lower lever on inhaler
- Wait at least 60 seconds before taking the next inhalation

Figure 4.2 Different inhaler devices and instructions for their use.

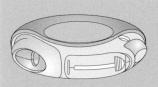

Accuhaler (Diskus)

- Hold the outer casing in one hand while pushing the thumb grip away until you hear a click

- With the mouthpiece towards you, slide the lever away until it clicks; this makes the dose available and moves the counter on

- Breathe out gently away from the mouthpiece, then put mouthpiece in mouth and breathe in

- Remove inhaler and hold your breath for 10 seconds

- Close by sliding thumb grip back towards you until it clicks

Diskhaler

To load:

- Remove mouthpiece cover; pull the tray out gently until you can squeeze the ridges on each side and slide it out

- Place the foil disk on the wheel, numbers upwards, and slide the tray back

- Hold the corners of the tray and slide it in and out to rotate the disk until the highest number (8 or 4) shows in the window

To use:

- Keeping the Diskhaler level, raise the rear of the lid as far as it will go so that the pin pierces the blister in the disk

- Still keeping the Diskhaler level, breathe out gently, put mouthpiece in mouth and breathe in as deeply as possible; do not block the two small air vents on the sides of the mouthpiece

- Remove Diskhaler from mouth and hold your breath for 10 seconds

- Slide tray in and out to prepare next dose

Pressurized metered-dose inhalers (pMDIs) have, hitherto, been the most widely used type of inhaler, but their use is declining in many countries because of concern about the environmental effects of the chlorofluorocarbons (CFCs) used as propellants. These inhalers deliver a measured dose of medication, and delivery is efficient when the device is used correctly (see Figure 4.1).

Many patients, however, are unable to coordinate inspiration with inhaler actuation. The use of a spacer device (Figures 4.3–4.5) can overcome this problem to some extent. The medication is discharged into the spacer and held in suspension for several seconds. During this time, the patient can inhale the drug in one or several breaths, without the need to coordinate inspiration and drug delivery; this may be particularly useful in small children and patients with poor coordination. A small-volume spacer can be adapted with a face mask for young children. The use of spacers also reduces oropharyngeal deposition of drug and the incidence of local side effects, and allows high doses to be given during attacks.

Inhalers containing 'ozone-friendly' propellants, such as hydrofluoroalkanes, have been introduced to replace the CFC-containing pMDIs. Dissolution of the topical corticosteroid beclometasone dipropionate in a hydrofluoroalkane leads to the release of smaller particles on activation of the inhaler, and thus improved drug deposition and efficacy. This increases systemic bioavailability from lung

(a)   (b)

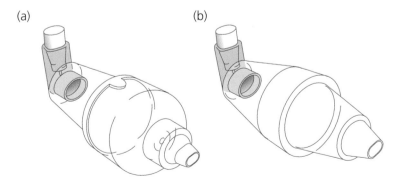

Figure 4.3 Spacer devices for use by (a) young children who need assistance and (b) patients who can use the device without help.

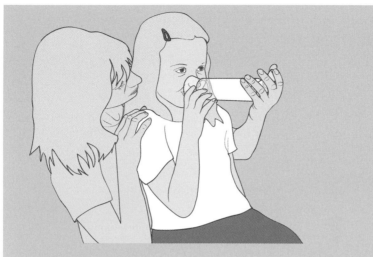

- Shake the inhaler and insert it into the spacer
- Put the mouthpiece into the child's mouth and seal the child's lips around the mouthpiece
- The child should breathe in and out slowly and gently
- Depress the canister as the child breathes in and out: one puff for at least every four breath cycles
- Remove the spacer from the child's mouth
- Generally, two puffs is adequate – this can be repeated every few minutes in acute severe asthma (see Chapter 5)

Figure 4.4 Use of a spacer by a young child – instructions for parents/carers.

absorption and consequently increases the risk of side effects unless the dose is adjusted accordingly.

Breath-actuated inhalers, in which the valve is actuated during inspiration, are useful in patients who have difficulty coordinating actuation and breathing. Drug deposition appears to be greater than with pMDIs. As with pMDIs, however, propellants are needed to discharge the drug.

Dry-powder inhalers (DPIs) require a different inhalation technique from that needed with pMDIs. No propellant is needed because the

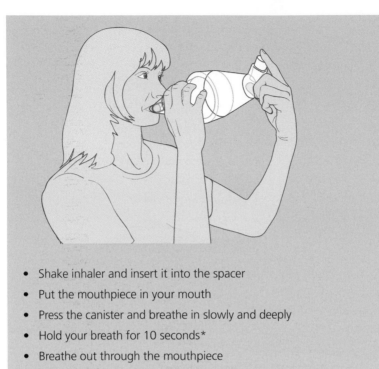

- Shake inhaler and insert it into the spacer
- Put the mouthpiece in your mouth
- Press the canister and breathe in slowly and deeply
- Hold your breath for 10 seconds*
- Breathe out through the mouthpiece
- Breathe in again, but do not press the canister this time
- Remove the device and wait for 30 seconds before taking another inhalation

*Alternatively, breathe normally through the spacer for at least four breaths.

Figure 4.5 Use of a spacer by a patient who can operate it without help.

drug is released by inspiratory airflow. However, a certain minimum flow rate is required, and thus these devices may be less effective in young children and during severe attacks. Inhalation of dry particles can cause coughing.

Nebulizers generate a wet aerosol by blowing compressed air through a drug solution or suspension, or by ultrasonic vibration. The patient inhales the aerosol through a face mask or mouthpiece. Nebulizers have largely been replaced in emergency settings and for young children by pMDIs and spacers, which have demonstrated equivalent drug delivery.

This removes the need to purchase a nebulizer and air pump, and avoids the problems of portability of this equipment in emergency or remote settings. Nebulized therapy is still used for those with very severe lung disease or extreme attacks. A standard dose of nebulized β_2-agonist is equivalent to 12–16 puffs from a pMDI and spacer.

Stepwise approach to asthma treatment

Current management guidelines recommend a stepwise approach to asthma treatment, depending on disease control (Table 4.5), in both adults and children (Figure 4.6). All patients should aim to have well-controlled asthma, and treatment should be stepped up or down, as appropriate, every 1–3 months to achieve and maintain asthma control.

TABLE 4.5

Levels of asthma control*

Symptom	Asthma		
	Well controlled	Partly controlled	Uncontrolled
Daytime symptoms	< twice a week	> twice a week	≥ 3 features of partly controlled asthma present in any week
Limitation of activities	None	Any	
Night-time symptoms	None	Any	
Need for rescue reliever treatment	< twice a week	> twice a week	
Lung function	Normal	< 80% predicted or personal best (if known)	
Exacerbation	None	≥ 1per year	

*From Global Initiative for Asthma slide set. www.ginasthma.org

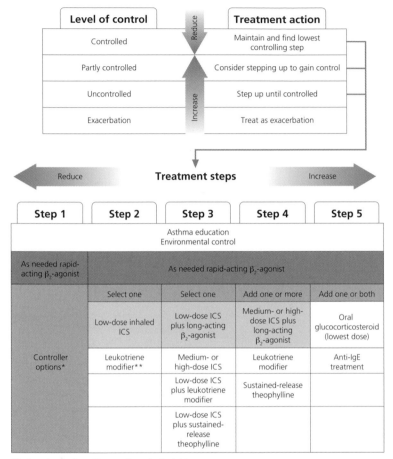

Level of control		Treatment action
Controlled	Reduce	Maintain and find lowest controlling step
Partly controlled		Consider stepping up to gain control
Uncontrolled	Increase	Step up until controlled
Exacerbation		Treat as exacerbation

Reduce ← **Treatment steps** → Increase

Step 1	Step 2	Step 3	Step 4	Step 5
	Asthma education Environmental control			
As needed rapid-acting β₂-agonist	As needed rapid-acting β₂-agonist			
	Select one	Select one	Add one or more	Add one or both
Controller options*	Low-dose inhaled ICS	Low-dose ICS plus long-acting β₂-agonist	Medium- or high-dose ICS plus long-acting β₂-agonist	Oral glucocorticosteroid (lowest dose)
	Leukotriene modifier**	Medium- or high-dose ICS	Leukotriene modifier	Anti-IgE treatment
		Low-dose ICS plus leukotriene modifier	Sustained-release theophylline	
		Low-dose ICS plus sustained-release theophylline		

*Preferred controller options are shown in shaded boxes
**Receptor antagonist or synthesis inhibitors

Alternative reliever treatments include inhaled anticholinergics, short-acting oral β₂-agonists, some long-acting β₂-agonists, and short-acting theophylline. Regular dosing with short- and long-acting β₂-agonist is not advised unless accompanied by regular use of an inhaled glucocorticosteroid.

Figure 4.6 Stepwise approach to the long-term management of asthma in children older than 5 years, adolescents and adults. Patients should start treatment at steps 2 or 3 depending on their levels of symptoms and indicators of asthma severity. A rescue course of prednisolone may be needed at any time and any step. ICS, inhaled glucocorticosteroids; Ig, immunoglobulin. Reproduced with permission from the Global Initiative for Asthma, 2008. *Global Strategy for Asthma Management and Prevention.* Available at www.ginasthma.org

Recommended management strategies suggest five treatment steps. Patients should be started on therapy appropriate to the initial level of symptoms: step 2 is appropriate for most patients who are receiving no, or only as-needed, bronchodilator treatment for asthma, and step 3 is appropriate for those with more uncontrolled symptoms and reduced lung function at the start of treatment.

Depending on symptom severity and the presence of exacerbations, treatment should be continued at a given level for 1–3 months before considering escalation or reduction. Generally, after 3 months of well-controlled asthma a step down to a lower level of treatment should be considered.

Step 1 is indicated for asthma with infrequent symptoms (less than twice a week) and normal interval lung function. For these patients, an inhaled as-needed SABA may be appropriate therapy without a regular controller treatment. Such patients can still experience exacerbations and the intensity of treatment for exacerbations should depend on the severity of the exacerbation (see Chapter 5).

Step 2 is usually indicated for initial treatment in those who have moderate symptoms. It involves the regular use of a low-dose inhaled corticosteroid medication in addition to a rapidly acting β_2-agonist for symptom relief as needed. The dose of inhaled corticosteroid at this level would range from 200 to 500 µg daily of beclometasone or equivalent medication in adults, and 100 to 200 µg daily in children. While the best available evidence supports inhaled corticosteroids for asthma treatment at this level for prevention of exacerbations and symptom control, leukotriene modifiers are an alternative at this treatment step. Leukotriene modifier medication is particularly favored in children for whom the dose of inhaled corticosteroid needs to be minimized, although existing evidence suggests that leukotriene modifier medication is less effective in preventing exacerbations than low-dose inhaled corticosteroid medication.

Step 3. Patients who still have symptoms of uncontrolled asthma despite using a low-dose inhaled corticosteroid, or those with more severe symptoms without treatment, should progress to step 3. This involves the addition of a LABA to regularly administered low-dose inhaled corticosteroid therapy and as-needed short-acting reliever therapy. The available evidence suggests that use of a LABA at this level provides symptom control superior to that from increasing doses of inhaled corticosteroids.

An alternative method of delivering therapy at this or later stages of management is a combined inhaled corticosteroid/LABA for both preventer and reliever therapy. This relies on the use of a rapid- and long-acting β_2-agonist (formoterol) in combination with a low-dose formulation of inhaled corticosteroid (usually budesonide, 200–400 µg twice daily) to be used as both controller and reliever therapy. This treatment has the advantage of convenience, as well as enabling the delivery of increased doses of inhaled corticosteroid for symptoms, thereby increasing anti-inflammatory controller treatment at the first sign of worsening symptoms. Evidence supports this approach for reducing asthma exacerbations. A potential concern with this approach is that patients may not take regular controller medication, and education therefore needs to emphasize the importance of using the budesonide/formoterol inhaler for both regular maintenance as well as reliever treatment.

At this treatment step, other options are the addition of a theophylline to low-dose inhaled corticosteroid medication or the addition of a leukotriene modifier, but both these treatment strategies appear to be less effective than the combination of a LABA with low-dose inhaled corticosteroid.

Step 4. Patients with more severe asthma and persistent symptoms despite step 3 treatment should be treated with escalating doses of inhaled corticosteroid and LABA therapy in addition to a SABA. Moderate to high doses of inhaled corticosteroid treatment are up to 2000 µg daily of beclometasone or equivalent in adults and up to 400 µg in children. At this level of treatment, additional controllers such as sustained-release theophylline or leukotriene modifiers can also be used.

Step 5. The highest level of treatment, step 5, involves the addition of oral corticosteroid treatment and/or anti-IgE therapy for patients with uncontrolled asthma despite the use of high-dose controller inhaled corticosteroids and LABAs. Such unresponsive asthma symptoms should prompt a consideration of the diagnosis of asthma and the exclusion of other factors that may be worsening asthma. It is also appropriate to seek specialist referral at this stage. Oral corticosteroids should be used at the lowest dose and for the minimum time required to gain asthma symptom control.

Infants and young children. The symptom-driven stepwise approach to asthma care described above is similar in children. Generally, in very young children, low-dose inhaled corticosteroid treatments are preferred at step 2 of care. The dose ranges of inhaled corticosteroids should be considerably lower for children than for adults. Children over 7 years of age can usually use a puffer and spacer device, while those under 4 years of age are likely to require a face mask and spacer to deliver asthma treatments effectively. Between these ages the choice of device depends on the child and their experience with the medication.

Written treatment plan. All patients with asthma should have a written plan that describes their current step of asthma treatment and advises on treatment adjustments to accommodate worsening asthma (see Chapter 6). For many patients, such a plan will also involve instructions to take oral corticosteroids or seek medical advice for prescription of oral corticosteroid treatment.

When recommended treatment fails

In the event of poor asthma control using medication recommended in guidelines, it is important not to escalate treatment without careful consideration of whether it is warranted. Three questions should be asked:

- Is the patient receiving the medication?
- Does the patient really have asthma?
- Does the patient have severe asthma?

Is the patient receiving the medication? Many obstacles exist to patients receiving their medication. The medication may be difficult to obtain for reasons of cost or inconvenience. It then has to be taken. Patients perform a 'cost–benefit' analysis as to whether to take the medication, an analysis that includes their beliefs about the benefits of the treatment and the likely outcome of their asthma, and their fears about side effects. The health professional must take part in this analysis and address issues that arise in order to aid adherence to a medication plan.

Patients then need to use their device effectively. Many people, especially the young and very old, find this difficult. A major part of consultation with a patient who is not successful in achieving good asthma control should be a review of inhaler use and technique, as this can be a significant barrier to effective treatment.

Does the patient really have asthma? Other diagnoses to consider are listed in Figure 3.2, page 41. Any patient who does not respond to medication should undergo lung function testing to confirm the diagnosis. Physical examination may suggest that other investigations, such as chest radiography, might be relevant. For children too young to perform spirometry reliably (usually under 7 years of age), a specialist opinion should be sought if the diagnosis is uncertain, as in children the consequences of unnecessary inhalation of corticosteroids (> 400 µg per day) can be significant.

Does the patient have severe asthma? A very few patients do have severe asthma that continues to be unstable despite demonstrated reliable medication use. Such people should be referred to specialist care as other pharmaceutical options are available. Long-term use of oral corticosteroids should be moderated by the use of steroid-sparing agents.

Key points – management

- Drugs used in the management of asthma can be classified as controllers (preventers) or relievers: controllers are taken daily on a long-term basis to control persistent asthma; relievers are used to rapidly reverse the bronchoconstriction and associated symptoms during acute attacks.
- Controllers (e.g. inhaled corticosteroids) are the mainstay of asthma therapy. Increased use of relievers (short-acting β_2-agonists) indicates inadequate disease control.
- Asthma therapy should be tailored to disease severity; current management guidelines recommend a stepwise approach to treatment.
- All patients with asthma should have a written asthma action plan.
- If recommended treatment fails, adherence and diagnosis should be re-examined before treatment is escalated.

Key references

The Childhood Asthma Management Program Research Group. Long-term effects of budesonide or nedocromil in children with asthma. *N Engl J Med* 2000;343:1054–63.

Clark TJH, Godfrey S, Lee TH, eds. *Asthma.* 4th edn. London: Hodder Arnold, 2000.

Gibson PG, Powell H, Wilson A et al. Self-management education and regular practitioner review for adults with asthma. *Cochrane Database Syst Rev* 2002;issue 3:CD001117. www.thecochranelibrary.com

Global Initiative for Asthma. *Global Strategy for Asthma Management and Prevention*, Updated 2008. Available at www.ginasthma.org

National Heart, Lung and Blood Institute. *Expert Panel Report 3: Guidelines for the Diagnosis and Management of Asthma.* Bethesda: NHLBI, 2007. www.nhlbi.nih.gov/guidelines/asthma

Scottish Intercollegiate Guidelines Network. *British Guideline on the Management of Asthma*, Guideline 101. Edinburgh: SIGN, 2008 (revised June 2009). www.sign.ac.uk/guidelines

reaction for some and it requires recognition and treatment in its own right.

Some medications, such as β-blockers – even in eye drops – may also be responsible for an acute exacerbation of asthma. Individuals with acetylsalicylic acid (ASA; aspirin)-sensitive asthma may have severe asthma after taking ASA or other non-steroidal anti-inflammatory drug (NSAID). NSAID reactions are most often described in individuals with non-allergic asthma who have nasal polyposis. Individuals with this type of asthma must avoid ASA and all NSAIDs.

Regular use of controller asthma medication substantially reduces, but does not completely eliminate, the risk of an acute asthma attack. Asthma exacerbations may occur in individuals with asthma who do not receive adequate controller treatment. All individuals who present with an acute exacerbation should be asked what controller treatment they are taking, and consideration should be given to introducing or adjusting regular maintenance medication in order to prevent such exacerbations in the future.

Recognizing a severe attack

It is important for patients and clinicians alike to recognize the signs of a severe asthma attack and know when to seek further help.

Patients can recognize a severe asthma attack by the frequency and severity of symptoms (Figure 5.1). Asthma symptoms that recur and require bronchodilator treatment more frequently than once every 4 hours are an indication of an attack that requires medical treatment. Most often, patients with a severe exacerbation of asthma describe their asthma as being 'out of control'. This is a clear sign that urgent help is needed. Patients may also monitor their peak expiratory flow (PEF). A measurement of 50% of predicted or less that does not respond promptly to bronchodilator treatment is an indication for seeking emergency help.

Clinicians should assess the severity of an acute attack of asthma according to Table 5.1. It is important to remember that asthma severity is classified according to the worst parameter.

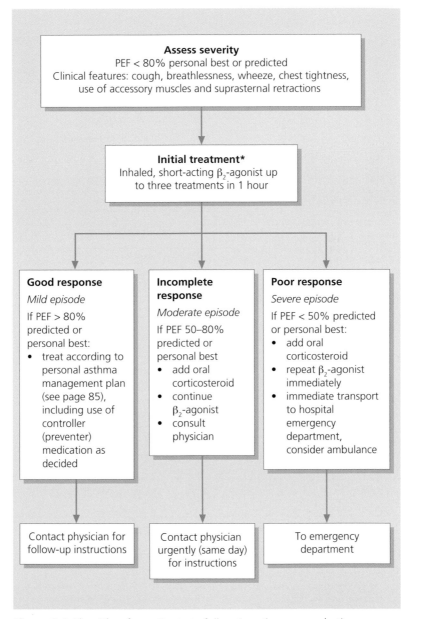

Assess severity
PEF < 80% personal best or predicted
Clinical features: cough, breathlessness, wheeze, chest tightness,
use of accessory muscles and suprasternal retractions

Initial treatment*
Inhaled, short-acting β_2-agonist up
to three treatments in 1 hour

Good response
Mild episode

If PEF > 80%
predicted or
personal best:
• treat according to
  personal asthma
  management plan
  (see page 85),
  including use of
  controller
  (preventer)
  medication as
  decided

**Incomplete
response**

Moderate episode

If PEF 50–80%
predicted or
personal best
• add oral
  corticosteroid
• continue
  β_2-agonist
• consult
  physician

Poor response
Severe episode

If PEF < 50% predicted
or personal best:
• add oral
  corticosteroid
• repeat β_2-agonist
  immediately
• immediate transport
  to hospital
  emergency
  department,
  consider ambulance

Contact physician for
follow-up instructions

Contact physician
urgently (same day)
for instructions

To emergency
department

Figure 5.1 Algorithm for patients to follow in asthma exacerbations.
*Patients at high risk of asthma-related death should contact a physician
promptly after initial treatment as additional therapy may be required.
PEF, peak expiratory flow.

TABLE 5.1

Classification of severity of asthma exacerbations

	Mild	Moderate
Breathless	When walking	When talking Infants: softer, shorter cry, difficulty feeding Can lie down
Speech: talks in...	Sentences	Phrases
Alertness	May be agitated	Usually agitated
Respiratory rate[†]	Increased	Increased
Accessory muscles and suprasternal retractions	Usually not	Usually
Wheeze	Moderate, often only end-expiratory	Loud
Pulse[‡]	< 100 bpm	100–200 bpm, depending on age
Pulsus paradoxus	Absent (< 10 mmHg)	May be present (unreliable) (10–25 mmHg)
PEF[§] after bronchodilator (% predicted or personal best)	> 80%	Approximately 60–80%
PaO_2 (on air)	Normal; test not usually necessary	> 60 mmHg
and/or $PaCO_2$	< 45 mmHg	< 45 mmHg
SpO_2 (on air)	> 95%	91–95%

Note: the presence of several signs, but not necessarily all, can be used to indicate the severity of an asthma exacerbation.
*Any of the listed features indicate a severe episode.
[†]Normal rates in children: < 2 months, 60 breaths/minute; 2–12 months, < 50 breaths/minute; 1–5 years, < 40 breaths/minute; 6–8 years, .< 30 breaths/minute.
[‡]Normal rates in children: 2–12 months, < 160 bpm; 1 year, < 120 bpm; 2–8 years, < 110 bpm.
[§]Children ≤ 7 years old and patients with very severe asthma are unlikely to be able to perform PEF readings.

Severe*	Respiratory arrest imminent
At rest Infants: stops feeding	
Prefers sitting	Hunched forwards
Words	
Usually agitated	Drowsy or confused
Often > 30 breaths/minute	
Usually	Paradoxical thoraco-abdominal movement
Usually loud but may become silent	Absent
> 120 bpm in adults 120–200 bpm in children, depending on age	Bradycardia
Often present (> 25 mmHg in adults, 20–40 mmHg in children)	Absence suggests respiratory muscle fatigue
< 60% (< 200 liters/minute in adults), or bronchodilator response lasts < 2 hours	
< 60 mmHg; possible cyanosis	
> 45 mmHg; possible respiratory failure	
< 90%	

bpm, beats per minute; $PaCO_2$, partial pressure of carbon dioxide in arterial blood; PaO_2, partial pressure of oxygen in arterial blood; PEF, peak expiratory flow; SpO_2, oxygen saturation estimated by pulse oximetry.

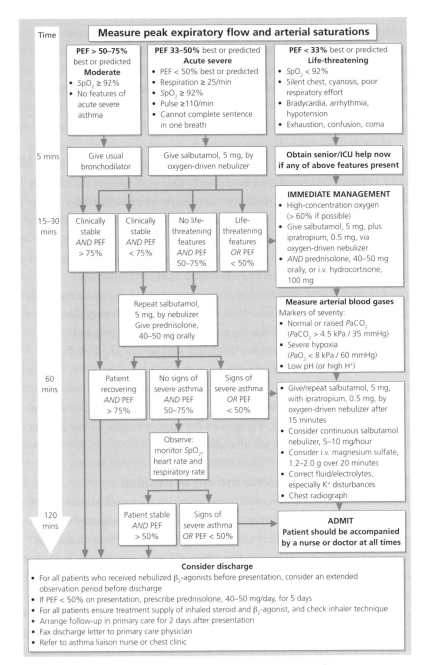

Figure 5.2 Acute asthma management in the emergency department.
Adapted from Scottish Intercollegiate Guidelines Network guideline, 2008.

All patients should receive inhaled bronchodilator, and those with moderate or severe exacerbations should receive oral or parenteral corticosteroid therapy. For patients with life-threatening attacks, intensive care services should be sought. Patients not responding to treatment and stable within 2 hours should be considered for admission to hospital.

In hospital. Acute asthma management in hospital is summarized in Figure 5.3. Once a patient is admitted to hospital, monitoring and treatment should continue with:
- frequent (at least every 2 hours) observation of PEF, oxygen saturation, blood pressure and pulse
- oxygen administration to maintain oxygen saturation above 92%
- administration of β_2-agonists at least every 4 hours, and continuously if required
- administration of corticosteroid therapy orally or intravenously
- observation for deterioration in clinical state.

For asthma exacerbations, 8–12 puffs of a β_2-agonist with a spacer device is approximately equivalent to 5 mg of salbutamol delivered by a nebulizer. In some instances, such as infection control or community use, this method of salbutamol delivery may be preferred.

Ongoing review in hospital ensures recovery and introduces patients to their ongoing preventative medication and the management plan likely to be required following a hospital admission for asthma. The time in hospital presents an ideal opportunity for formal asthma education; interventions that provide in-hospital asthma education have shown benefits in terms of reduced re-admission rates.

Follow-up

All patients should leave hospital with medication, a written plan of what to do if their asthma worsens and a follow-up medical appointment for ongoing management. Oral corticosteroid therapy should be continued for at least 5 days following discharge. It is important that asthma control is assessed following a hospital admission and that ongoing maintenance medication is adjusted accordingly.

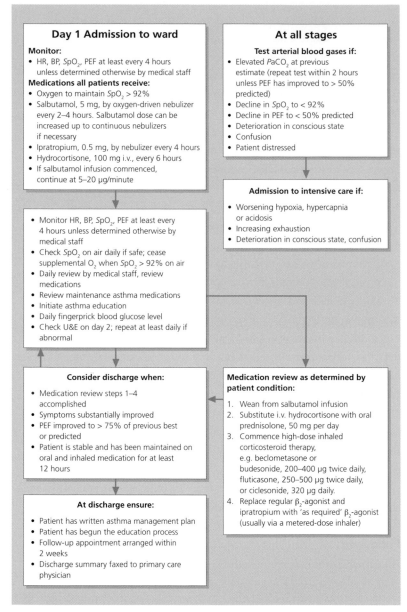

Figure 5.3 Algorithm for management in the hospital ward of adults with acute asthma. BP, blood pressure; HR, heart rate; $PaCO_2$, partial pressure of oxygen in arterial blood; PEF, peak expiratory flow; SpO_2, oxygen saturation estimated by pulse oximetry; U&E, urea and electrolytes.

Key points – acute asthma attacks

- Asthma exacerbations are one of the major causes of morbidity in asthma, resulting in loss of work time in adults or school absence in children, and emergency hospital presentation and admission.
- Causes of acute asthma include viral respiratory infections, acute allergen exposure, food allergies and some medications such as acetylsalicylic acid and non-steroidal anti-inflammatory drugs.
- Acute exacerbations of asthma usually respond well to inhaled β_2-agonists and a course of oral corticosteroid.
- After hospital admission, patients should receive appropriate medication, a written plan of what to do if their asthma worsens and a follow-up medical appointment for ongoing management and measurement of lung function.

Key references

Goeman DP, Aroni RA, Sawyer SM et al. Back for more: a qualitative study of emergency department reattendance for asthma. *Med J Aust* 2004;180:113–17.

Global Initiative for Asthma. *Global Strategy for Asthma Management and Prevention*, Updated 2008. Available at www.ginasthma.org

Scottish Intercollegiate Guidelines Network. *British Guideline on the Management of Asthma*, Guideline 101. Edinburgh: SIGN, 2008 (revised June 2009).
www.sign.ac.uk/guidelines

Preventing asthma attacks is the most effective means of controlling asthma. Effective prevention involves identifying and avoiding risk factors and asthma triggers, together with effective patient education and adherence to a medication regimen.

Patient partnerships

Included in the goals of good asthma management is the need to meet patients' goals and expectations as well as those of the health practitioners. Good asthma management means that a partnership should be established between the patient and health professional, with shared treatment goals noted in a jointly written and agreed self-management plan. This eases the pressure on healthcare personnel resources by helping patients to take responsibility for their health and improves asthma outcomes.

Risk factor avoidance

Identifying the risk factors that trigger asthma attacks and removing the appropriate allergens and irritants from the patient's environment can reduce the frequency of symptoms and hospitalizations for asthma, and the need for medication. Appropriate avoidance behaviors are shown in Table 6.1. However, allergens should only be avoided when there is evidence that the patient is indeed allergic to that specific allergen. Patients with a true allergy will have both a history of symptoms on exposure to an allergen and immunologic evidence of sensitivity, for example a positive skin-prick test or blood-specific immunoglobulin (Ig)E test. If these are not present then allergen avoidance is not recommended.

House dust mites are the most common source of domestic allergens. They breed fastest in damp humid climates. Avoidance measures should be particularly directed at the patient's bedroom, but ideally the entire home should be treated. Bed linen and blankets should be washed

TABLE 6.1

Allergen and irritant avoidance

Allergen avoidance

House dust mite

- Wash bed linen and blankets once a week in hot water (> 55°C)
- Protect mattresses and pillows with air-tight covers
- Remove carpets, particularly in bedrooms
- Avoid fabric-covered furniture
- Wash curtains and soft toys
- If possible, use a vacuum cleaner with filters

Animal allergens

- Remove animals from house
- If removal of family pets is not possible or desirable, keep animals out of bedrooms and wash the animal regularly

Cockroach allergen

- Clean infected houses regularly
- Use pesticides (but ensure asthmatic patient is not present if pesticide sprays are used, and air house thoroughly before patient returns)

Fungal spores and pollens

- Close doors and windows and remain indoors when mold and pollen counts are highest
- Air conditioning can be helpful providing the unit is kept clean

General measures

Tobacco smoke

- Stop smoking
- Avoid smoking in rooms used by children with asthma
- Avoid public areas where people smoke

CONTINUED

TABLE 6.1 (CONTINUED)

Indoor air pollutants
- Vent all furnaces and stoves to exterior
- Keep rooms well ventilated
- Avoid household sprays and polishes

Colds and other viral respiratory infections
- Patients with asthma should have annual influenza vaccination
- When cold symptoms appear, treat with inhaled short-acting β_2-agonist, introduce oral corticosteroids early, or increase inhaled corticosteroid dose if asthma status deteriorates
- Continue anti-inflammatory treatment for several weeks to ensure adequate control

Physical activity
- Should not be avoided, but appropriate medication is necessary:
  - pretreat with short- or long-acting β_2-agonist or cromoglicate before exercising
  - training and warm-up exercises can reduce symptoms

weekly in hot water, and mattresses and pillows protected by air-tight covers. Carpets and furnishing fabrics should be avoided wherever possible, and the bedroom should be well ventilated. Acaricides are of little use. Unfortunately, even with these measures it is difficult to reduce the concentrations of domestic mite allergens below the threshold that induces symptoms in allergic individuals.

Animal allergens. A pet in the home to which the patient with asthma is allergic is a major risk factor for current asthma symptoms. Ideally, such pets – usually cats – should be removed from the home, but this may not be acceptable. If animals cannot be removed, they should be kept away from bedrooms; weekly washing of the pet appears to reduce the allergen load but may be poorly tolerated by the animal.

Cockroach allergen is a major cause of asthma in some areas. It can be reduced by regular cleaning of the home and by the use of pesticides.

If pesticide sprays are used, however, the patient should not be present while spraying is in progress, and the home should be aired thoroughly before the patient returns.

Molds and pollens. The number of fungal spores can be reduced by removing or cleaning mold-infested objects. A low humidity (less than 50%) is important, and so a dehumidifier or air conditioning may be useful; such devices should be cleaned regularly. Exposure to outdoor allergens, such as pollens, can be minimized by keeping doors and windows closed, and by remaining indoors as much as possible during high-risk periods.

Smoking. Passive smoking increases the risk of allergic sensitization in children and worsens the frequency and severity of symptoms in asthmatic children. Parents of such children should be advised not to smoke and to prohibit smoking in rooms used by their children.

Indoor pollutants. Common indoor pollutants include nitrogen dioxide, carbon monoxide and particles. Adequate ventilation and maintenance of heating systems are the most effective measures for reducing exposure to such pollutants.

Occupational exposure. Early identification of occupational sensitizers and removal of the patient from further exposure are important elements in the management of occupational asthma.

Food allergy is a rare cause of asthma exacerbations and may occur at any age. Individuals with severe food allergies should avoid the food in question and be assessed by an allergy specialist. Clear evidence of IgE immunoreactivity to the food or a positive double-blind food challenge should be obtained to justify and clarify the role of ongoing food avoidance. Patients with both asthma and severe food allergies causing anaphylaxis are at particular risk of early death. They should be well educated in the avoidance of the specific food and should have access to injectable epinephrine (adrenaline).

Acetylsalicylic acid (ASA) intolerance is an important cause of worsening asthma in adults. Patients who are affected should be advised to avoid all non-steroidal anti-inflammatory drugs (NSAIDs) except those selective against cyclooxygenase-2 (COX-2) inhibitors.

Treatment of rhinitis

Symptoms of rhinitis include a runny, itchy or blocked nose and there may also be sneezing and symptoms of eye irritation and tiredness. Rhinitis is more common than asthma, and international surveys reveal that its prevalence appears to be increasing. The prevalence of asthma is increased in those with both allergic and non-allergic rhinitis by two- to fivefold, and 80% of individuals with asthma suffer from symptoms of rhinitis. It is increasingly evident that effective treatment of rhinitis can assist in the management of asthma. Regular use of topical nasal corticosteroids is the recommended treatment for all but mild intermittent rhinitis. Topical nasal corticosteroid therapy for rhinitis in those with concurrent asthma in addition to regular controller asthma therapy can nearly halve the risk of asthma exacerbations requiring emergency treatment. Allergen immunotherapy can also be an effective treatment for severe or refractory allergic rhinitis, and an associated improvement in asthma outcomes has been shown.

Immunotherapy

Specific immunotherapy, aimed at treating the underlying allergy, has been shown to be effective in patients with asthma caused by house dust mite, grass or other pollens, animal dander or *Alternaria sp*. Such treatment may be useful in patients for whom allergen avoidance is not possible or whose symptoms are poorly controlled by conventional medication. Allergen immunotherapy is usually delivered by the subcutaneous route by a medical practitioner. However, there is increasing evidence to support the use of sublingual immunotherapy. As immunotherapy is relatively contraindicated in those with unstable asthma and those with abnormal lung function, it is practically limited to those with milder disease, especially those who suffer from allergic rhinitis. There is some evidence that immunotherapy can prevent the progression of allergic rhinitis to asthma.

Immunotherapy should only be undertaken by healthcare professionals with specific training in the diagnosis of allergy and the management of anaphylaxis.

Asthma management plans

Education is essential to enable patients to make the decisions needed to control their asthma. This involves the preparation of a detailed management plan (Table 6.2), which is agreed between the patient and the physician, and is tailored to the needs and circumstances of the individual patient. Plans based on symptoms and on peak expiratory flow (PEF) have been shown to be equally effective. Plans should be written down so patients can refer to them (Figures 6.1 and 6.2).

A zone system, which classifies the level of asthma control according to symptoms and PEF (if available), is a useful feature of management plans. This approach helps patients to understand the chronic and variable nature of asthma, monitor their condition, identify signs of deteriorating control and take appropriate action.

TABLE 6.2

Elements of an asthma management plan

- The daily dose of long-term preventive medication needed to control asthma and prevent symptoms

- Specific triggers to avoid

- What to do if asthma worsens:

  - name and dose of bronchodilator to be taken immediately for quick relief of symptoms

  - how to recognize deteriorating control (e.g. increasing cough, chest tightness or breathing difficulties, nocturnal symptoms, increasing use of quick-acting reliever medicine)

  - how to treat worsening asthma, and what to do if a cold develops

  - how and when to seek medical attention

Traffic-light plan. In the management plan shown in Figure 6.1, the three zones correspond to the colors of a traffic light.

The green zone indicates 'all clear'. Asthma is controlled, with few symptoms (less than two a week) and no interference with everyday life; PEF is 80–100% of personal best and PEF variability is less than 20%. Moving to a lower treatment step can be considered if the patient remains in this zone for at least 3 months.

The yellow zone indicates that caution is necessary. Mild symptoms are present and PEF is 60–80% of personal best with 20–30%

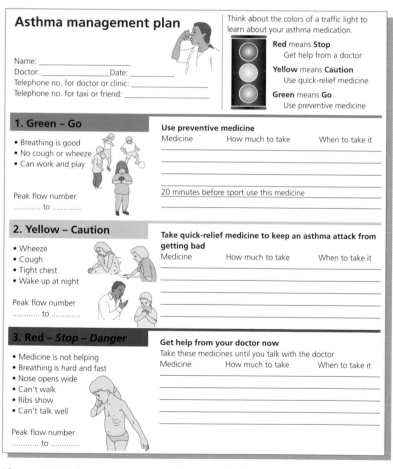

Asthma management plan

Think about the colors of a traffic light to learn about your asthma medication.

Name: _____
Doctor: _____ Date: _____
Telephone no. for doctor or clinic: _____
Telephone no. for taxi or friend: _____

Red means **Stop**
　Get help from a doctor
Yellow means **Caution**
　Use quick-relief medicine
Green means **Go**
　Use preventive medicine

1. Green – Go

- Breathing is good
- No cough or wheeze
- Can work and play

Peak flow number
.... to ....

Use preventive medicine

Medicine　　　How much to take　　　When to take it

20 minutes before sport use this medicine

2. Yellow – Caution

- Wheeze
- Cough
- Tight chest
- Wake up at night

Peak flow number
.... to ....

Take quick-relief medicine to keep an asthma attack from getting bad

Medicine　　　How much to take　　　When to take it

3. Red – *Stop – Danger*

- Medicine is not helping
- Breathing is hard and fast
- Nose opens wide
- Can't walk
- Ribs show
- Can't talk well

Peak flow number
.... to ....

Get help from your doctor now
Take these medicines until you talk with the doctor
Medicine　　　How much to take　　　When to take it

Figure 6.1 Asthma management plans can be based on a zone system, with action needed to control asthma at different levels of severity.

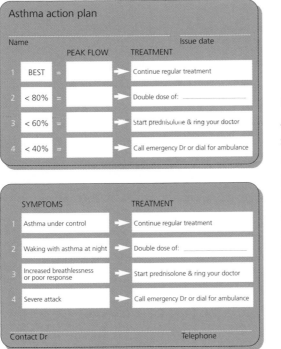

Figure 6.2
A credit-card-sized asthma self-management plan. This plan has been evaluated in clinical trials and introduced in several countries.

variability. This may indicate an acute attack requiring a temporary increase in medication, or an overall deterioration that requires additional treatment.

The red zone indicates an emergency. Asthma symptoms are present at rest and may interfere with activity; PEF is below 60% of personal best. Immediate intervention is necessary.

Credit-card-sized plan. Another management plan, the credit-card-sized document shown in Figure 6.2, has been evaluated in clinical trials, and has been successfully introduced in several countries, including the UK, New Zealand and Australia.

Promoting adherence. Patients' asthma will not be controlled effectively if they do not adhere to their medication and management plan, yet adherence studies reveal that fewer than 50% of patients take their medication as prescribed. Causes of non-adherence may or may not be related to medication (Table 6.3).

Regular consultations are necessary to give patients an opportunity to talk about their concerns, needs and expectations in relation to their asthma and its treatment. Action can then be taken to address any problems identified, and to resolve any fears or concerns that patients may have. Strategies for encouraging adherence are listed in Table 6.4. Together, the patient and the healthcare professional can identify joint

TABLE 6.3

Factors leading to non-adherence with asthma therapy

Medication-related factors

- Misunderstanding the need for both long-term and short-acting drugs
- Complicated treatment regimens
- Difficulty in giving medicine to young children
- Difficulty using inhalers
- Adverse effects
- Fear of adverse effects or addiction
- Cost
- Dislike of medication
- Distance to pharmacies

Non-medication factors

- Disbelief or denial of cause of symptoms or attacks
- Misunderstanding of management plan
- Lack of guidance for self-management
- Dissatisfaction with healthcare professionals
- Fears or concerns not expressed or discussed
- Inappropriate expectations
- Poor supervision, training or follow-up
- Cultural issues (traditions, beliefs about asthma and its treatment)
- Family issues (e.g. smoking, pets)

TABLE 6.4

Strategies for improving adherence to asthma treatment

- Enquire about adherence to medication (patients are generally honest in admitting non-adherence)
- Educate patients and their families about the inflammatory basis of asthma and the need for ongoing treatments
- Enquire about and address concerns regarding medications and their use
- Identify and, if possible, address barriers to medication use (e.g. cost, knowledge of how to use the devices)
- Ask about family and cultural beliefs
- Encourage the patient in self-management
- Keep medication regimens simple – twice a day maximum
- Plan for reminders to use medication such as alarms, mobile phones
- Explain likely side effects and how to prevent them
- Be positive about the outcomes of treatments
- Plan for regular medical review at least twice a year

goals of treatment, such as 'staying out of hospital', 'attending school camp' or 'playing football', that are relevant to the patient and therefore likely to promote adherence. At each visit, the physician should check:

- whether the stated goals have been achieved
- adherence to, and concerns about, medication and the management plan
- the patient's use of the controller (preventer) and reliever inhalers, PEF meter or other devices
- need for emergency attendances
- avoidance of triggers.

Once control has been achieved, regular follow-up every 1–6 months is necessary to assess whether the management plan is meeting its objectives. This includes an assessment of asthma control, including:

- nocturnal symptoms
- the effect of symptoms on normal activity
- use of reliever rescue medication

89

- need for urgent medical attention
- spirometry or peak flow reading.

When to refer

In general, most patients with mild or moderate asthma can be adequately managed in the primary care setting. Referral to a specialist is advisable for patients with moderate or severe persistent asthma, those reaching step 5 of the GINA management guideline and those with complicating conditions or circumstances (Table 6.5). Children needing more than 400 µg inhaled beclometasone (beclomethasone) or the daily equivalent of inhaled corticosteroid, and adults needing more than 1000 µg per day with poor symptom control, should also be referred to a specialist.

TABLE 6.5

Situations requiring specialist referral for asthma

- Life-threatening attacks
- Moderate or severe persistent asthma
- Patient is unable to cope with self-management
- Atypical signs or symptoms, or difficulties with differential diagnosis
- Complicating conditions such as sinusitis, nasal polyposis, aspergillosis or severe rhinitis
- Further diagnostic tests required (e.g. provocation testing or complete lung function tests)
- Patient does not respond optimally to treatment
- Additional guidance needed (e.g. trigger avoidance or treatment complications)

Key points – preventing asthma attacks

- Preventing asthma attacks is the most effective means of controlling asthma.
- Identifying risk factors that trigger asthma attacks and removing the appropriate allergens and irritants from the patient's environment can reduce the frequency of symptoms and hospitalizations for asthma, and decrease the need for medication.
- Immunotherapy is helpful in some patients when one of the following applies:
  - specific allergens can be shown to be causative
  - allergen avoidance is not possible
  - symptoms are not controlled by conventional medication.
- A written self-management plan empowers patients to manage their asthma optimally.
- Failure to respond to treatment may result from non-adherence to the prescribed treatment. Attention must be paid to the patient's ability to take their inhaled therapy correctly.
- Adherence to medications is a major challenge to healthcare practitioners and patients. Identifying problems surrounding care and creating a patient partnership with agreed treatment goals can facilitate adherence.

Key references

Abramson MJ, Puy RM, Weiner JM. Allergen immunotherapy for asthma. *Cochrane Database Syst Rev* 2003;issue 4:CD001186. www.thecochranelibrary.com

Allergic Rhinitis and its Impact on Asthma. www.whiar.org

Gibson PG, Powell H, Wilson A et al. Self-management education and regular practitioner review for adults with asthma. *Cochrane Database Syst Rev* 2002;issue 3:CD001117. www.thecochranelibrary.com

Global Initiative for Asthma. www.ginasthma.org

Powell H, Gibson PG. Options for
self-management education for adults
with asthma. *Cochrane Database
Syst Rev* 2002;issue 3:CD004107.
www.thecochranelibrary.com

Exercise-induced asthma

Up to 80% of people with asthma will develop exercise-induced symptoms, so that exercise for some people is a noticeable trigger for asthma. Indeed, in some people asthma is only evident on exercising; this is particularly the case for children, in whom the benefits of exercise are especially important. Consequently, managing exercise-induced asthma and enabling individuals to exercise despite asthma is an important part of asthma management.

In addition, the issue of asthma in elite sporting activities has risen to prominence. In some Olympic teams as many as 20% of athletes declare that they have asthma, raising concerns about the appropriate use of anti-asthma medications in this group. Optimizing asthma diagnosis and treatment in elite athletes is critical to optimizing performance and deserves particular attention.

Diagnosis

Exercise-induced asthma is defined as a transient increase in airway resistance that follows vigorous exercise. Many people complain of shortness of breath while exercising, and this symptom is often magnified in people with asthma. Typically, people with asthma describe developing wheeze, shortness of breath and sometimes cough both during and, more importantly, after exercise. For some individuals with brittle asthma, the response to exercise can be severe and may be a strong disincentive to exercise.

Exercise-induced asthma appears to be more common in those with allergies to inhaled substances and often occurs on exercise in very cold weather. A feature is a refractory period, whereby induction of exercise-induced asthma appears to be protective for further episodes for a period of several hours. Thus, individuals who experience a bout of exercise-induced asthma can undertake subsequent exercise with relative protection from further episodes. This refractory period can be inhibited by anti-inflammatory medications such as indometacin.

In the laboratory or for research, exercise-induced asthma can be brought on by a short period (6–8 minutes) of high-intensity exercise of at least 70% of maximum predicted capacity. Lung function is measured following this exercise; a decline in the forced expiratory volume in 1 second (FEV_1) of more than 10% from baseline denotes a diagnosis of exercise-induced asthma (Figure 7.1).

The problem with laboratory exercise tests is that they may not replicate the environmental conditions under which exercise is performed; for example, neither the temperature nor the humidity of ambient air is likely to be the same as that encountered during outdoor exercise. In addition, it is often difficult to achieve adequately high workloads for very fit individuals such as athletes using laboratory exercise equipment. Hence, field testing can be undertaken to make the diagnosis, which requires recording of peak expiratory flow (PEF) or lung function following exercise in the field. However, this too is subject to varying conditions of humidity, temperature and conduct of the test, rendering standardization difficult. As a consequence of these difficulties, surrogate challenges for exercise-induced asthma have been developed.

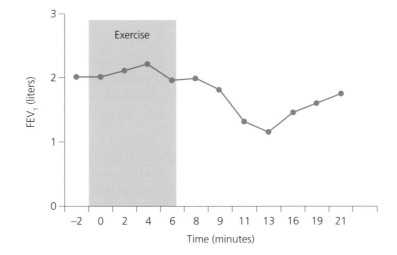

Figure 7.1 Exercise challenge testing: during brief high-intensity exercise, lung function transiently improves, but lung function is likely to fall in the minutes following exercise in people with exercise-induced asthma.

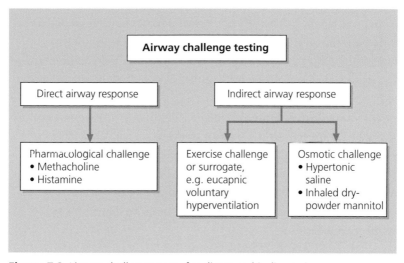

Figure 7.2 Airway challenge tests for direct and indirect airway responses.

Airway challenge testing can be categorized into direct and indirect airway responses (Figure 7.2). Indirect challenges cause bronchoconstriction by stimulating airway mast cells to release mediator and thereby cause secondary airway smooth muscle constriction. Direct challenges act pharmacologically on the airway smooth muscle to cause airway narrowing.

Indirect challenges. Exercise challenge testing is an indirect challenge relying on airway responses to exercise, such as airway drying and cooling, to cause smooth muscle contraction. Because of the difficulties of replicating field exercise in the laboratory to achieve consistency of diagnosis, a number of surrogate challenges for exercise have been developed. Chief among these is the eucapnic voluntary hyperventilation challenge, in which the individual is asked to breathe a mixture of dry air with 5% carbon dioxide at 85% of their maximal ventilation (approximately 30 times FEV_1) for 6 minutes, and their FEV_1 is monitored after challenge. This surrogate challenge has been shown to correlate very well with actual exercise challenge and is suitable for use by athletes. A fall in FEV_1 of 10% following the eucapnic voluntary hyperventilation challenge has been adopted by the International Olympic Committee as the preferred criterion for confirmation of an asthma diagnosis in elite athletes.

95

Indirect airway challenges such as mannitol and hypertonic saline have been shown to correlate very well with eucapnic voluntary hyperventilation challenges. These agents mimic the dehydration of the airways that is probably responsible for exercise-induced asthma (see 'Mechanisms', below).

Direct challenges. Most individuals with airway hyperresponsiveness to methacholine will yield a positive result to exercise challenge. However, some – particularly elite – athletes will have a positive surrogate exercise challenge result despite negative direct airway challenge test results. It is therefore important not to exclude exercise-induced asthma on the basis of a negative direct airway challenge test result.

Mechanisms

During inhalation air is humidified and warmed to body temperature. At rest, this process usually occurs in the upper airways, particularly in the nose. During exercise, ventilation is increased, sometimes to levels exceeding 100 L/min, so that the individual has to breathe through the mouth to overcome upper airway resistance. Mouth breathing and increased ventilation lead to recruitment of the lower airways to warm and humidify inspired air, resulting in progressive evaporation of airway surface fluid and hyperosmolarity of this fluid. It is thought that hyperosmolarity of the airway surface fluid provokes mast cell degranulation, which can then stimulate airway narrowing through smooth muscle contraction. In support of these theories, exercise-induced asthma has been shown to correlate with increased blood mast cell mediators. In addition, breathing humidified warmed air during exercise has been shown to be protective for the development of exercise-induced bronchoconstriction. Swimming is often recommended as exercise to people with asthma, as inspiration will occur from the humidified air near the water surface, decreasing the dehydrating stimulus to the lower airways.

By contrast, many individuals with asthma find cold air a potent trigger of symptoms. This is because the water content of air is temperature dependent, cold air holding less water than warmer air. Thus, exercise in the cold, such as skiing, requires greater water transfer for complete saturation of inspired air than does exercise in warmer climates, and cold dry air is therefore a more potent stimulus for developing exercise-induced asthma.

Exercise-induced symptoms appear to be more common in atopic individuals; this observation may imply that inhaled allergens play a role. In particular, loss of the protective functions of the upper airways during inspiration may permit increased penetration to the lower respiratory tract of allergens and other particles likely to stimulate asthma. Although this has not been proved to be a cause in laboratory-induced exercise-induced asthma, increased lower airway exposure to allergens and extremes of environmental changes such as heat and cold may be particularly relevant in elite athletes who spend a large amount of time training with high ventilation, thereby increasing their cumulative exposure to such potential triggers.

Exercise-induced asthma in athletes

The high prevalence of exercise-induced asthma in elite athletes is a recently recognized problem. Escalating use of bronchodilator treatments by elite athletes has prompted rulings from the International Olympic Committee. Some elite cold-weather athletes, such as cross-country skiers, will develop exercise-induced asthma (so called 'skier's asthma'). In summer athletes, a high occurrence of asthma has been reported in elite swimmers. In both these instances, training for prolonged periods at high ventilatory workloads and consequent large exposure to very cold or chlorinated air, respectively, is thought to contribute to an airway injury that may lead to exercise-induced asthma. The finding that older athletes and those from sports that are predominantly aerobic are more likely to have exercise-induced asthma supports this theory.

The symptoms of elite athletes with asthma are thought to differ from those of non-athletes in that they may complain of poor performance or fatigue rather than dyspnea. Investigation of symptoms of elite athletes revealed that traditional asthma symptoms have a sensitivity of only 60% in predicting exercise-induced bronchoconstriction in laboratory challenge. Thus, poor performance in an athlete ought to prompt consideration of exercise-induced asthma.

The diagnosis of exercise-induced asthma in elite athletes must be verified by airway challenges. Eucapnic voluntary hyperventilation and mannitol are both suitable challenges for this purpose.

Treatment

Treatment for exercise-induced asthma in those with pre-existing asthma is determined by evaluating lung function and symptoms. Individuals with lung function abnormalities and symptoms of asthma both with and without exercise should have the usual controller (preventer) medication prescribed. Inhaled corticosteroids have been shown to be very effective in reducing airway hyperresponsiveness both generally and following exercise. However, many people with asthma do have asthma symptoms despite regular use of inhaled corticosteroids and may require additional short-acting β_2-agonists (SABAs) before exercise to prevent exercise-induced asthma.

Some individuals with normal interval lung function complain of symptoms only on exercise. Although regular preventive treatment may be appropriate for such people if exercise is very frequent, it may be reasonable to use SABAs to prevent exercise-induced bronchoconstriction in those who experience symptoms only episodically, such as less than twice a week. Additional or alternative treatments may be required in some, and include mast cell stabilizers such as cromoglicate or nedocromil, or leukotriene modifiers such as montelukast.

Non-drug strategies for the treatment of exercise-induced asthma rely on the refractory period that follows induction of airway narrowing with exercise. It is frequently recommended that athletes with exercise-induced asthma warm up slowly. They may institute strategies such as repeated high-intensity runs during a warm-up to prevent exercise-induced asthma occurring in the main competition.

Key points – exercise-induced asthma

- Exercise-induced asthma is defined as a transient increase in airway resistance that follows vigorous exercise.
- It appears to be more common in those with atopy and to be seen more often on exercise in very cold weather.
- Induction of exercise-induced asthma appears to be protective for further episodes for a period of several hours.
- Exercise testing or other direct or indirect challenges are used in diagnosis.
- In elite athletes, direct airway challenges may not reveal exercise-induced asthma, so indirect surrogate challenges must be used to confirm diagnosis.
- First-line treatment of exercise-induced asthma is inhaled corticosteroids to reduce airway hyperresponsiveness, with additional short-acting β_2-agonists before exercise if necessary.

Key references

Fitch KD, Sue-Chu M, Anderson SD et al. Asthma and the elite athlete: summary of the International Olympic Committee's Consensus Conference, Lausanne, Switzerland, January 22–24, 2008. *J Allergy Clin Immunol* 2008;122:254–60.

Holzer K, Anderson SD, Douglass J. Exercise in elite summer athletes: Challenges for diagnosis. *J Allergy Clin Immunol* 2002;110:374–80.

Immunologic treatments

The incidence of allergy and asthma in developing countries has increased with the acquisition of westernized lifestyles. It has been suggested that this observed increase may be due to the decreasing incidence of childhood infections and other environmental influences such as alteration in diet and intestinal bacterial flora. Immune stimulation by infections in early life may be necessary for the differentiation of T regulatory lymphocytes which can modulate immune responses. Observations that a rural lifestyle appears to offer some protection from allergic diseases may support this theory.

Studies are under way to attempt to manipulate the responses to allergens early in life to facilitate the development of regulatory immune responses. These include trials of mycobacterial vaccines and probiotics.

Allergen immunotherapy is a productive area for future developments. Some evidence exists that allergen immunotherapy can prevent the development of asthma in those with allergic rhinitis and may also prevent new sensitizations to inhaled allergens. Increasing attention is being devoted to the development of safer forms of injected allergen immunotherapy and more convenient modes of sublingual administration of allergen immunotherapy extracts.

Other therapeutic approaches

Other therapies that look promising in the management of chronic severe asthma include:

- biological agents that block the effects of tumor necrosis factor (TNF)-α (e.g. soluble TNF-α receptor or monoclonal antibodies that can block TNF-α)
- selective antagonists for chemokine receptors (CCR), especially CCR3, which is involved in the recruitment of mast cells and eosinophils into the inflamed airways
- selective type-4 phosphodiesterase inhibitors, which have an anti-inflammatory action on a variety of inflammatory cells implicated in

asthma pathogenesis and additionally exert some effect in relaxing airway smooth muscle
- ketolide antibiotics to treat asthma exacerbations: effectiveness may reflect anti-infective or anti-inflammatory effects
- monoclonal antibodies that reduce eosinophil numbers in the airways and hence exacerbation rates in those with severe eosinophilic asthma.

In addition, intensive research is focused on developing a safer form of inhaled corticosteroid that interferes with the inflammatory pathways underpinning the pathogenesis of asthma and yet does not produce the usual side effects.

Bronchial thermoplasty uses heat to diminish the amount of airway smooth muscle and therefore reduce bronchial hyperresponsiveness. While early reports appear positive, evidence of long-term outcome is awaited.

Assessing airway inflammation

The development of methods of measuring the underlying airway inflammation in asthma heralds changes in the choice of asthma treatments. The most commonly used non-invasive method of establishing the nature of airway inflammation is induced sputum analysis for cells, which is cumbersome to incorporate into daily clinical practice. The refinement of this and other methods of quantifying airway inflammation – such as measurement of exhaled gases, particularly exhaled nitric oxide – may be more convenient and allow more precise direction of treatments.

Genetic targeting

As treatments become more geared towards total prevention and cure of asthma, it is likely that they will focus not on broad populations, but on individuals who are at specific genetic risk. Identifying asthma susceptibility genes is almost a growth industry at present. Although certain genes that increase the risk either of having asthma or of having more severe disease have been identified, it is likely that many more will be found that are more important and are, therefore, of direct relevance in selecting patients for appropriate treatments.

The results of genetic studies are also likely to have an impact on drug treatment, as polymorphisms involving cellular receptors or enzyme pathways against which drugs are directed may influence their effectiveness (pharmacogenetics).

The future looks most promising for patients with asthma but, until new treatments are developed, it is essential that we make better use of the drugs currently available.

Key references

Barnes PJ. Cytokine-directed therapies for the treatment of chronic airway diseases. *Cytokine Growth Factor Rev* 2003;14:511–22.

Blease K, Lewis A, Raymon HK. Emerging treatments for asthma. *Expert Opin Emerg Drugs* 2003; 8:71–81.

Bush RK. The use of anti-IgE in the treatment of allergic asthma. *Med Clin N Am* 2002;86:1113–29.

Erin EM, Williams TJ, Barnes PJ, Hansel TT. Eotaxin receptor (CCR3) antagonism in asthma and allergic disease. *Curr Drug Targets Inflamm Allergy* 2002;1:201–14.

Grootendorst DC, Rabe KF. Selective phosphodiesterase inhibitors for the treatment of asthma and chronic obstructive pulmonary disease. *Curr Opin Allergy Clin Immunol* 2002;2:61–7.

Haldar P, Brightling CE, Hargadon B et al. Mepolizumab and exacerbations of refractory eosinophilic asthma. *N Engl J Med* 2009;360:973–84.

Useful resources

UK

Asthma UK
Summit House, 70 Wilson Street
London EC2A 2DB
Tel: +44 (0)20 7786 4900
Helpline: 0800 121 62 44
info@asthma.org.uk
www.asthma.org.uk

British Lung Foundation
73–75 Goswell Road
London EC1V 7ER
Tel: +44 (0)20 7688 5555
Helpline: 08458 50 50 20
www.lunguk.org

British Thoracic Society
17 Doughty Street
London WC1N 2PL
Tel: +44 (0)20 7831 8778
bts@brit-thoracic.org.uk
www.brit-thoracic.org.uk
Scottish Intercollegiate Guidelines
Network (SIGN)
www.sign.ac.uk/guidelines/fulltext/
101/index.html

National Asthma Campaign
Providence House, Providence Place
London N1 0NT
Tel: +44 (0)20 7226 2260
Helpline: 08457 01 02 03

USA

**Allergy & Asthma Network
Mothers of Asthmatics**
2751 Prosperity Ave, Suite 150
Fairfax, VA 22031
Tel: 1 800 878 4403
www.aanma.org

**American Academy of Allergy,
Asthma & Immunology**
555 East Wells Street, Suite 1100
Milwaukee, WI 53202
Tel: +1 414 272 6071
info@aaaai.org
www.aaaai.org

**American Association for
Respiratory Care**
9425 N MacArthur Blvd
Suite 100, Irving, TX 75063
Tel: +1 972 243 2272
info@aarc.org
www.aarc.org

American Lung Association
1301 Pennsylvania Ave. NW
Washington, DC 20004
Tel: +1 202 785 3355
Helpline: 1 800 586 4872
www.lungusa.org

Asthma and Allergy Foundation of America
8201 Corporate Drive, Suite 1000
Landover, MD 20785
Toll-free: 1 800 727 8462
info@aafa.org
www.aafa.org

US Environmental Protection Agency
www.epa.gov/asthma

International
Allergic Rhinitis and its Impact on Asthma
www.whiar.org

The Asthma Foundation (New Zealand)
Level 1, Panama House
22 Panama Street, PO Box 1459
Wellington 6140
Tel: +64 (0)4 499 4592
info@asthmafoundation.org.nz
www.asthmanz.co.nz

The Lung Association (Canada)
1750 Courtwood Crescent, Suite 300
Ottawa, ON, K2C 2B5
Tel: +1 613 569 6411
Toll-free: 1 888 566 5864
info@lung.ca
www.lung.ca

European Academy of Allergy and Clinical Immunology
Tel: +41 44 205 55 33
info@eaaci.net
www.eaaci.net

European Federation of Allergy and Airway Diseases Patients' Association
Tel: +32 (0)2 227 2712
info@efanet.org
www.efanet.org

Global Initiative for Asthma
www.ginasthma.org

International Union Against Tuberculosis and Lung Disease
Tel: +33 (0)1 44 32 03 60
www.theunion.org

National Asthma Council Australia
Suite 104, Level 1, 153–61 Park St.
Melbourne, VIC 3205
Tel: +61 (0)3 9929 4333
Toll-free: 1 800 032 495
nac@nationalasthma.org.au
www.nationalasthma.org.au

Thoracic Society of Australia & New Zealand
145 Macquarie Street, Sydney
NSW 2000, Australia
Tel: +61 (0)2 9256 5457
admin@thoracic.org.au
www.thoracic.org.au

Index

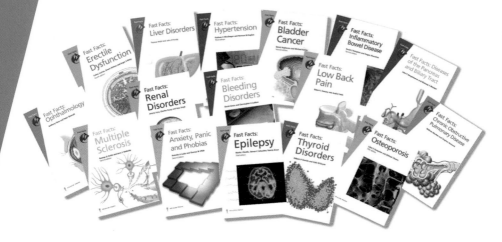